Centerville Library
Washington-Centerville Public Library
Centerville, Ohio
DISCARD

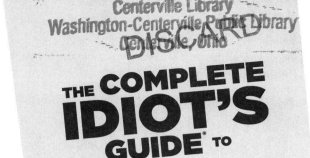

W9-BSZ-409

Pilates on the Mat

by Karon Karter

ALPHA

A member of Penguin Group (USA) Inc.

Centerville Library
Washington-Centerville Public Library
Centerville, Ohio

This book is dedicated to my devoted mother, whom I love more than life itself, and Janet Harris, my writing coach, who continues to mold and shape my writing career.

ALPHA BOOKS

Published by the Penguin Group

Penguin Group (USA) Inc., 375 Hudson Street, New York, New York 10014, USA • Penguin Group (Canada), 90 Eglinton Avenue East, Suite 700, Toronto, Ontario M4P 2Y3, Canada (a division of Pearson Penguin Canada Inc.) • Penguin Books Ltd., 80 Strand, London WC2R 0RL, England • Penguin Ireland, 25 St. Stephen's Green, Dublin 2, Ireland (a division of Penguin Books Ltd.) • Penguin Group (Australia), 250 Camberwell Road, Camberwell, Victoria 3124, Australia (a division of Pearson Australia Group Pty. Ltd.) • Penguin Books India Pvt. Ltd., 11 Community Centre, Panchsheel Park, New Delhi—110 017, India • Penguin Group (NZ), 67 Apollo Drive, Rosedale, North Shore, Auckland 1311, New Zealand (a division of Pearson New Zealand Ltd.) • Penguin Books (South Africa) (Pty.) Ltd., 24 Sturdee Avenue, Rosebank, Johannesburg 2196, South Africa • Penguin Books Ltd., Registered Offices: 80 Strand, London WC2R 0RL, England

First edition originally published as *The Complete Idiot's Guide to the Pilates Method.*

Copyright © 2012 by Karon Karter

All rights reserved. No part of this book shall be reproduced, stored in a retrieval system, or transmitted by any means, electronic, mechanical, photocopying, recording, or otherwise, without written permission from the publisher. No patent liability is assumed with respect to the use of the information contained herein. Although every precaution has been taken in the preparation of this book, the publisher and author assume no responsibility for errors or omissions. Neither is any liability assumed for damages resulting from the use of information contained herein. For information, address Alpha Books, 800 East 96th Street, Indianapolis, IN 46240.

THE COMPLETE IDIOT'S GUIDE TO and Design are registered trademarks of Penguin Group (USA) Inc.

International Standard Book Number: 978-1-61564-147-5
Library of Congress Catalog Card Number: 2011912284

14 13 12   8 7 6 5 4 3 2 1

Interpretation of the printing code: The rightmost number of the first series of numbers is the year of the book's printing; the rightmost number of the second series of numbers is the number of the book's printing. For example, a printing code of 12-1 shows that the first printing occurred in 2012.

Printed in the United States of America

Note: This publication contains the opinions and ideas of its author. It is intended to provide helpful and informative material on the subject matter covered. It is sold with the understanding that the author and publisher are not engaged in rendering professional services in the book. If the reader requires personal assistance or advice, a competent professional should be consulted.

The author and publisher specifically disclaim any responsibility for any liability, loss, or risk, personal or otherwise, which is incurred as a consequence, directly or indirectly, of the use and application of any of the contents of this book.

Most Alpha books are available at special quantity discounts for bulk purchases for sales promotions, premiums, fund-raising, or educational use. Special books, or book excerpts, can also be created to fit specific needs.

For details, write: Special Markets, Alpha Books, 375 Hudson Street, New York, NY 10014.

Publisher: *Marie Butler-Knight*
Associate Publisher: *Mike Sanders*
Executive Managing Editor: *Billy Fields*
Executive Acquisitions Editor: *Lori Cates Hand*
Senior Development Editor: *Christy Wagner*
Senior Production Editor: *Kayla Dugger*

Copy Editor: *Amy Lepore*
Cover Designer: *Kurt Owens*
Book Designers: *William Thomas, Rebecca Batchelor*
Indexer: *Tonya Heard*
Layout: *Ayanna Lacey*
Proofreader: *John Etchison*

ALWAYS LEARNING   PEARSON

Contents

Introduction

Rather than sucking in your gut and wishing you looked svelte in your little black dress, try Pilates. It's a whole-torso workout that strengthens your abs and back and also straightens your posture, making you feel taller. Pilates combines the allure of rebalancing your mind as you fine-tune your body from head to toe. Joseph Pilates' prophecy sums it up nicely: in 10 sessions, you'll feel the difference; in 20, you'll see the difference; in 30, you'll have a new body.

Whether you want to expand your Pilates knowledge or try it for the first time, you've come to the right place.

How This Book Is Organized

The book is divided into three parts:

Part 1, Live in Your Body, explains why you should join the Pilates movement. As you read on, you'll learn about the muscles that support your frame and keep you standing tall. Plus, you'll discover why your breath can enhance your life.

Part 2, Show Me the Mat, introduces you to Mat exercises in the correct sequence and to core concepts so you can get the body you deserve. These exercises are the same ones taught by Joseph Pilates. Before long, you'll move just like he did!

I wrote **Part 3, Moving On Up,** with two goals in mind: to challenge you and to give you enough exercises for a lifetime. In this part, you learn the advanced Mat exercises, plus the Side-Kick Series and the Standing Arms Series.

A Little Something Else

This book also contains a few easy-to-recognize sidebars that offer inspirational quotes from Joseph Pilates as well as tips, definitions, and extra information to help you along the way. Keep an eye out for the following elements to enhance your knowledge:

DEFINITION

These sidebars contain words or common lingo used in Pilates. Lengthen your lingo, and you're on your way to perfecting your Pilates.

FIT FACT

These sidebars are home to tips and tidbits about Pilates that may be helpful to know while you practice.

ON THE MAT

For inspirational quotes from Joseph Pilates, along with historical information, read these sidebars.

PILATES PRECAUTION

Heed these warnings to prevent getting into a sticky situation.

Acknowledgments

Yes, I dreamed it and put my thoughts to words to invent this book. However, this enormous task couldn't have been accomplished without so many gracious people.

A very special thanks to Toni Beck, the 50-plus coordinator and researcher for the Baylor/Tom Landry Sports Medicine and Research Center in Dallas, Texas. She defies her age with grace and beauty.

A thank you debt I'll never be able to return extends to my graphic designer, Bo Mikolajczyk. He stayed up with me all night to design the pictures for this book the way I wanted them.

Thank you to City Lights of San Francisco, my favorite workout clothes, for providing me with some great-looking outfits for the pictures in this book. And a special thanks goes to Kristin Moses (she just had a baby 6 months prior to the shoot and looks great—thanks to Pilates) for modeling and allowing me to shoot the pictures in this book in her studio, Perform Studio.

Hugs and kisses to MGB—thank you for your emotional support and patience during the months of this project.

I'm grateful for the entire team at Alpha Books, who massaged my words even more to make this a great book. Many thanks for keeping me moving toward my passion.

My family is great because they continue to support me during the ups and downs of my writing career.

I can't leave without giving Colleen Glenn a special thank you. She taught me Pilates; her certification program is the best one out there! But that's not all. Thank you so much, Colleen, for your emotional support and for sharing your expertise with me while I wrote this book.

Trademarks

All terms mentioned in this book that are known to be or are suspected of being trademarks or service marks have been appropriately capitalized. Alpha Books and Penguin Group (USA) Inc. cannot attest to the accuracy of this information. Use of a term in this book should not be regarded as affecting the validity of any trademark or service mark.

Live in Your Body

Part 1 introduces you to your frame and the muscles that support your "center" and keep you standing tall. You also learn about your breath and how good breathing techniques enhance your life.

In short, this part gets you ready for the chapters to come and helps you heighten your life for the better.

Join the Movement

In This Chapter

- Pilates 101
- Getting to know your body
- Introducing Joseph Pilates
- Pilates for all walks of life

Would you believe me if I told you there's a workout that can give you longer, leaner legs plus to-die-for buns without weight-room bulk? What if I also told you this same workout gives you a firmer, flatter midsection and improves your posture, and it can also make you taller and feel more energized? Would you still believe me? Now imagine the unthinkable: you actually look forward to this workout.

Keep reading, because all this and more is waiting for you. It's called Pilates.

Introducing Pilates

Joseph Pilates (1880–1967; pronounced *puh-LAH-teez*) is the visionary behind this promising workout. Pilates is a total body-conditioning workout for both men and women that engages your body and leaves you refreshed and alert with an enormous amount of self-confidence. It's an intense, ongoing challenge, blending Eastern and Western philosophies of physical and mental conditioning.

Pilates gives you the stretching benefits of yoga along with the great muscle tone of a nautilus workout. It focuses on muscular harmony and balance and is a whole new way to get your body moving.

But don't take my word for it. Here are some testimonies from some of my students, who share their reasons for taking and loving Pilates. See where you fit in:

"After participating in a Mat class for less than a year, I have found my abdominal muscles to be stronger than in any other form of exercise I've done for more than 20 years. Because of this abdominal toning paired with very concentrated and controlled breathing patterns, my spine has become much more flexible and my posture more erect. Pilates has helped improve the quality of other forms of exercise such as yoga and weight lifting. I only wish I had begun studying it years ago." —Sandra Roberdeau

"What Pilates has done for me is elongate my muscles; I look leaner just by using my own body weight for resistance. I do so many other forms of exercise—kickboxing, running, aerobics, spinning, and weight training. However, with Pilates, I feel I am getting just as much of a 'workout' and am being gentler and kinder to myself. And I do the Mat exercises right in my hotel room while I travel for my job, which I do half the month." —Penny Pollack

"Pilates is an escape for me from the daily rush. It is the only time of the day that I concentrate on myself. I always feel good for the rest of the day after a class and actually feel taller! Having three children (twins and two C-sections), I look forward to my classes with Karon for both mental and physical conditioning." —Wendy Poston

"After two back surgeries, my physical therapist recommended Pilates. I have been exercising with the Mat for over a year now, and my back feels great. In fact, my posture is better, I feel taller, and I am more flexible and stronger than ever. By strengthening those 'core' muscles, the stabilizing muscles, I am able to do everything I did before back problems and do them better." —Kurt Liese

 ON THE MAT

In the words of Joseph Pilates, "The Prophecy: in 10 sessions, you'll feel the difference; in 20, you'll see the difference; and in 30, you'll have a whole new body."

The Pilates workout changes how you feel about your body. It increases your vitality, makes you feel years younger, and improves your posture while toning those "flabby" muscles. Furthermore, the Pilates system eliminates most nagging back pain, and your sex life will improve because you'll function better in those vital areas. Plus, you'll love your body.

The Thinking Body

Pilates creates a thinking body. I'm sure you're familiar with the five senses—sight, smell, hearing, taste, and touch. But you also get information from various inner senses that make up your *proprioceptive system*, which literally means "own reception."

DEFINITION

Your **proprioceptive system,** which literally means "own reception," coordinates every movement you make. These exercises are designed to get you to know your body.

This system is sort of an internal dialogue that feeds you information to eat, to drink, to stop, to go, etc. Deep within you, this system communicates information about your body that no one else is privy to. Proprioception coordinates your every movement; it enables the pianist to place his fingers in the right place without looking or the quarterback to know instinctively when to take the ball and run with it. The mind has an innate way of controlling your muscles so they perform what you want, how you want.

The exercises designed by Joseph Pilates require concentration and precision of movement. With practice and repetition, you'll fine-tune your proprioceptive sense and learn to focus mentally. Eventually, your body will execute these moves, no matter how demanding, with precision, control, and fluidity of motion without you having to think about what you're doing. Joseph Pilates called his method "Contrology" because it was designed to teach exercisers how to gain the mastery of their minds over the complete control of their bodies.

To be sure, some exercises are difficult. Your legs may quake, and you may hear the voice in your head saying, *Give up. This is too hard.* But don't listen!

These moves pinpoint imbalances in your body, whether it's lack of strength, coordination, flexibility, balance, or muscular imbalances. Everyone has weaknesses, but with practice and repetition, these moves get easier as your mind tells your body what to do. Accomplishing this feat proves that you can do more for yourself—and your life. Pushing yourself when you think *I can't* is a gift to yourself—and that's empowering.

Perseverance stays with you long after the workout. You'll learn to live in your body and have a certain level of awareness about yourself. You'll learn to embrace your imbalances, find ways to overcome them, accept yourself a little better, and like your body a little more because you didn't give up—that's self-discipline.

FIT FACT

Self-discipline means regulating oneself for the sake of self-improvement, which is what Joseph Pilates espoused and embodied!

When you're mentally in tune with what you're doing, you become physically alert; the mind controls the body. These exercises can help you achieve this heightened level of well-being—to live in your body.

Body Therapy

Over the last few decades, thanks to so much of the population becoming couch potatoes and eating a poorer and poorer diet, we've witnessed a dramatic shift in our bodies. They've gone south, right? This immobility ruins our bodies. Besides flabby muscles, movement in our joints becomes rusty.

Yet it's not too late to get your body in motion! To stop this decay, you need to strengthen and stretch your body. You know there are no shortcuts to a better body, so you must get your body off the couch. How about learning to use your body, but not in an out-of-breath, heart-pounding sweat session?

The exercises in this book are more subtle. As you grow with movement, you'll learn things about your body, particularly its imbalances. You'll also learn how to listen to your body—you know, those subtle aches and pains and hidden quirks.

Ever get frustrated because you can't do what you used to do at 20? With a little more wear and tear on our bodies, most of us can't move like we used to. We get tighter as we age. Is that so bad, though? If we didn't grow older, we would stay stagnant, emotionally and physically. Pilates teaches you to grow; an aging body doesn't have to deteriorate.

Embrace your weaknesses so you'll learn how to live in harmony with your body, young or old. Joseph Pilates' methods, in a sense, keep you moving forward.

Do you live with chronic pain—perhaps a stiff lower back, a popping knee, or an achy shoulder? You live with these and other hidden stresses every day. Your body has learned to cope with them. Many students claim that only after training in Pilates did they realize that they've been living with chronic pain. For example, minor back pains. Have you ever stopped to think why your back aches? Could it be from movements you take for granted?

Your everyday movements might take a toll on your body. Instead of moving through life in an out-of-control, jerky manner, use Joseph's methods, which teach controlled moves and no traumatic movements. This control will spill over into your everyday life. As you become more aware of your body and how it functions, you are more likely to live a healthier life.

With these exercises, you'll increase flexibility, improve balance and coordination, build strength, and tone muscles—it's a resistance workout without all that bulk. These exercises can also help you improve your posture, rejuvenate your energy level, relieve stress, and reduce fatigue and chronic pain. Within every exercise, you'll work on the following:

- Flexibility

- Strength

- Balance

- Coordination

Pilates offers a complete connection between body and mind; it's a feel-great workout because you don't have to run yourself ragged to get in shape.

ON THE MAT

Here is Joseph Pilates' 1945 definition of the ideal physical fitness: "The attainment and maintenance of a uniformly developed body with a sound mind fully capable of naturally, easily, and satisfactorily performing our many and varied daily tasks with spontaneous zest and pleasure."

By accomplishing the exercises described in this book, you can take a time-out from the daily pressures of life, have a quiet session for your mind, and get rid of the body blues. You'll feel good about your body as you witness a little shift in flab composition and gain a tremendous amount of self-confidence—and, in doing so, you'll create a new, happier you.

The Man Behind the Method

Joseph Pilates was a legendary body healer. His own sickly childhood made him passionate about ways to combat sickness through conditioning and strengthening the body. In fact, asthma and other childhood ailments didn't keep him from becoming an accomplished gymnast, boxer, diver, and skier.

He admired the Eastern traditions of mindful body conditioning, particularly its focus on calmness, freeing the mind, and being centered and whole, with an emphasis on stretching. In addition, he mastered the Western approach to Greek and German fitness that emphasized strength and muscle tone. Joseph combined the two to develop his own mind and body workout.

Joseph had an opportunity to experiment with his principles during World War I. He invented exercise apparatus for inactive patients by attaching springs to their hospital beds. He invented ways to exercise their limbs, stretch their spines, and develop their core strength while they were bedridden. In fact, he used anything he could get his hands on—his bunk, the bedsprings, and a chair, for example. This inspiration was the prototype of several pieces of equipment used today. At that time, his vision was just a concept. Today, however, you'll see this equipment in most studios, plus the real heart of his work, the Mat workout.

What was amazing, given such distressed surroundings, is that Joseph's methods worked. Because he was so successful at getting his patients moving, he was asked to train the most elite armed forces of the British military. After that, performers and many athletes turned to Joseph for hard-core training. For example, Max Schmelling, the famous heavyweight boxing sensation, relied on Joseph to train him.

Of course, behind every great man there's a woman. Clara Pilates was devoted to her husband and his work; she was a nurse whom he met while emigrating from Germany to live the American dream. In 1926, they opened their first studio in New York City at 939 Eighth Avenue and taught Joseph's vision of ideal fitness. The Pilates movement is about 90 years older than most traditional exercise programs.

ON THE MAT

In a 1959 interview, Joseph Pilates said, "Movements are planned to relieve the heart, lungs, and liver of constriction caused by modern day living …."

Your Inner Athlete

Chances are you've heard of Pilates, but maybe you're really not sure what to expect or even if you can do this workout. Anyone can do Pilates, and your fitness level doesn't matter. Pilates can be your primary mode of body conditioning and injury prevention, or you can supplement it with your own weekly exercise routine. That was Joseph's dream—a workout that anyone and everyone can use, from basic to advanced levels of fitness, from the injured to the super-fit, at any age and any level of ability.

You won't sweat to loud music, nor will you pound the pavement to achieve great muscle tone. You won't lift anything heavier than a set of 5-pound dumbbell weights.

Instead, Pilates is based on six extremely sound principles:

- Concentration
- Control
- Centering
- Flow
- Precision
- Breathing

The routines are biomechanically safe and nonimpact. The moves stretch and strengthen all the major muscle groups without neglecting the smaller, weaker muscles.

There are two ways to work your body: a group Mat class or an individually instructed lesson using the apparatus invented by Joseph Pilates. You can do both. Each Mat class is specifically designed to work your muscles in a logical sequence. Some of the names given to these moves sound more like a game of Twister—the Teaser, the Boomerang, the Rollover. A typical Mat class lasts about an hour and costs about $10 to $25 per class.

If you decide to train on the specially designed equipment, don't feel intimidated by the medieval-looking machines equipped with leather straps, springs, and a trapeze. Keep in mind that this equipment was designed more than 90 years ago and delivers body results—an uplifted derriere, flat-ripped abs, and sleek, slender legs. It could be the only real anticellulite solution.

FIT FACT

Joseph invented more than 500 specific exercises on the following machines to develop the body uniformly: the Universal Reformer, the Cadillac, the Wunda Chair, the Electric Chair, the Spinal Corrector, the Ladder Barrel, the Ped-a-Pole, and the Magic Circle.

Don't fret—you won't be doing many repetitions. In other words, you won't crunch your heart out for sleek abs. Joseph preferred fewer, more precise movements requiring proper control and form. A typical workout will last an hour and, depending on the teacher, can cost about $50 to $100 per session.

The Achy Breaky Body

Pilates is now getting a fair amount of respect from the rehabilitative community. Physical therapists, chiropractors, and orthopedic surgeons around the world have included Pilates as part of their rehabilitative programs. For example, millions of people suffer from back pain—whether it's from poor posture, repetitive on-the-job action, or injury. The hallmark of Pilates is that each exercise addresses the spine. If done correctly, Pilates can alleviate most minor back pain.

> **PILATES PRECAUTION**
>
> If you have or had a back or knee injury, you should begin your reconditioning on the apparatus with the supervision of a teacher, preferably one who specializes in Pilates-based programs or a physical therapist trained in Pilates.

The rumor was, Joseph could fix your body. Dance legends such as Martha Graham, Ruth St. Denis, and George Balanchine flocked to Joseph's studio to make his discipline part of their training. He was popular because he rehabilitated an array of physical problems, from aching backs to knees—and keep in mind that physical therapy then was not the sophisticated science it is today. His methods simply worked!

Many of those dancers were able to resume their professional dancing careers. Still, a handful of them returned to New York to study with Joseph and Clara after they retired. In fact, these master teachers kept the "movement" alive and vibrant. These devotees dedicated their lives to teaching and spreading Joseph's ideas. Today, his exercises continue to thrive for both their recondition and fitness qualities mainly because his methods can be used by people in all walks of life!

Granny Got Her Groove Back

According to statistics, people today are living on average about 80 years. That is, provided healthful eating and regular exercise are part of the equation.

By exercising, you can protect against the development of high blood pressure, heart disease, cancer, depression, and osteoporosis. Exercise also can prevent disability and dependency, combat stress, and help you battle the bulge and sleepless nights.

Hundreds of research studies exist to prove it—in fact, exercise can do more than just about anything known to medical science to ensure a fit, healthy, and happy life. Pilates can safeguard your body and mind and help you age gracefully.

FIT FACT

Did Joseph Pilates invent the fountain of youth? Perhaps. He lived a long life—87 years. His devoted wife, Clara, lived into her mid-80s as well. They both dedicated their lives to teaching the ideal fitness program in their New York studio.

Stay Stronger Longer

You're as young as you feel. However, staying young at heart requires a commitment from you. Whether you're 20 or 50, it's never too late to start an exercise program to grow old with.

Changes in your health and appearance are a normal part of aging, but you don't have to surrender. You can slow the aging process by eating the right foods and exercising. Wasted muscles happen because of lack of activity, not old age. Here's a fact: an active person decreases $\frac{1}{2}$ percent physiologically per year, whereas an inactive or unfit person decreases 2 percent per year. Wasted muscles, a condition call *atrophy*, don't happen because of aging but because we don't get off the couch.

DEFINITION

Atrophy is a condition in which muscles waste away to the point you can't engage in day-to-day activities. This doesn't happen because of old age but because of an inactive, sedentary lifestyle. In fact, according to the American College of Sports Medicine (ACSM), 250,000 deaths in the United States per year are attributed to physical inactivity.

Inactivity affects how you live from day to day. It causes disease. If you continue to lose muscle fibers, the muscle will lose size and strength.

Stay stronger longer! By exercising, you increase your odds of staying independent with the freedom to move and get about. With Pilates, you can slow but not stop the age-related loss in muscle size and tone, as well as prevent poor posture. You can build strong muscles and develop balance in your hips, legs, and ankles so you can do activities that require quick movements. Imagine managing your own life into your 80s.

Exercise is critically important in your golden years. A research study showed that men and women age 90 and older increased their muscle strength more than 100 percent from lifting weights. Not only did they get stronger, but they were also able to walk better and take better care of themselves, according to the book *Fitness After 50; It's Never Too Late to Start*, written by Walter H. Ettinger Jr., MD, Brenda S. Mitchell, PhD, and Steven N. Blair, PED.

Battling Brittle Bones

Your bones are alive and kicking—in fact, your bones are continually remolding. You can influence how your bone remolds itself by exercising and eating well.

Your bones are made up of collagen and calcium. Collagen is a gluelike matter made up of vitamin C and water and helps form the structures of the body: skin, bones, teeth, blood vessels, cartilage, tendons, and ligaments—in short, the body's connective tissues. Calcium is a mineral that's stored in the bones so it can be used whenever it's needed for many vital body functions.

As the bones give up calcium, new bones are then molded. The body always needs calcium, so it pulls it from your bones, even if the supply is low. This deficit, then, affects how your bones are remade. Eating a diet high in calcium is your first line of defense.

FIT FACT

According to the Kaiser Institute on Aging, the body's metabolic rate drops about 2 percent per decade. After age 35, you'll have an increase in body fat and a decrease in bone density at a rate of 1 percent per year. You'll suffer more postural changes and a loss of connective tissue.

As you age, your bone production slows; your bones lose the ability to reshape new bones. Over time, the bones lessen in density and become thin, brittle, and susceptible to fractures. This decay is caused by both the natural aging process and a disease called osteoporosis. Osteoporosis accelerates loss of bone tissue, making bones brittle. Signs of osteoporosis can be as subtle as rounded shoulders or as severe as a hump in the upper back. This hump, called a dowager's hump, affects 40 percent of the women who have osteoporosis.

The good news is, the rate of bone loss can be slowed by regular resistance training. Yes—Pilates! The equipment utilizes springs to give you resistance, whereas you use your body as resistance during the Mat workout. In other words, Pilates gives you the same results as a weight-training program does. Study after study shows that walking and resistance training can slow the rate of bone loss, which helps prevent fractures and changes in posture. In addition to exercise, be sure you get good amounts of calcium and, in women, use estrogen-replacement therapy after menopause.

FIT FACT

Women have less bone mass to start with than men. During menopause, the ovaries stop producing estrogen, which protects against bone loss. After 50, bone loss in women starts to accelerate. Osteoporosis is the leading cause of bone fractures in the older population, causing an estimated 1.5 million fractures a year in the United States.

The best thing you can do in your 20s, 30s, and 40s is to build your bones early in life. A diet high in calcium and plenty of Pilates can help.

A Pea in a Pod

Pregnancy is kick-back and slack-off time—except when it comes to your body. After all, your body is about to change: more dimples, more stretch marks, more fat on the spots you've worked so hard to tone.

What you need at this time in your life more than anything else is lots of pampering: flowers, gifts, romantic dinners, and passionate kisses from the guy who put you in this temporary state of big belly. Still, you can give yourself and your baby the best gift: good health.

Pilates provides the perfect combination. It prepares your body for pregnancy by keeping your abs and pelvic muscles strong, keeping them flexible and toned while you're carrying your little bundle of joy. It also helps you get your body back after delivery. Nine months of pregnancy is nothing compared to reviving your bod!

Is It for You?

Your body, your mind, and your soul all experience a series of ups and downs during pregnancy—more downs, perhaps, than ups. Some women glow from head to toe; others can't lift their head out of the toilet bowl. Swelling, constipation, backache, fatigue, bloating, varicose veins, and nausea are common woes. Can Pilates help? You bet.

Regular exercise during pregnancy can help overcome some of the more difficult physiological and emotional changes—that is, if you're able to get out of bed. These exercises can reduce many of the annoying aches and pains of pregnancy, but is Pilates for you?

You might be looking for an exercise program that's nonimpact and tones your body. You've heard good things about Pilates: it strengthens the abs, tones the body, and doesn't put much stress on the body. All are true. So maybe you're thinking, *Great, I'll do these exercises while I'm pregnant.*

Know this: Pilates is not an exercise program you should try for the first time during pregnancy. The exercises may seem like a good choice during pregnancy, but you're strengthening muscles that in many cases haven't been used before, especially your abdominal and back muscles, and you're creating extra stress by trying a method that's quite complex. However, if you're shopping around several months *prior* to pregnancy, then Pilates is a good choice.

Taking charge of your health is empowering—it's good for you if you're planning ahead. If so, here's why these exercises can keep you healthy during and after your pregnancy:

- The exercises help develop strong abdominal muscles *before you get pregnant* and maintain them during pregnancy, two of the biggest gifts you can give yourself.

- Strong abs support a growing fetus.

- The exercises strengthen your back muscles, which can relieve lower-back pain from carrying the extra weight in your belly.

- The exercises keep your pelvic floor muscles toned for delivery and help you get them back after delivery.

- The movements are controlled—no jerky moves to put you at risk of over-stretching your ligaments and joints.

- The exercises prepare you for breath work.

PILATES PRECAUTION

Pilates is a great maintenance program during your pregnancy only if you have been practicing Pilates prior to your pregnancy. It's not advised to start Pilates after you become pregnant. Consult with your medical doctor or care provider before exercising during pregnancy.

Listen to the Doctor's Orders

As with any exercise program, use common sense. If you're planning to get pregnant, talk to your doctor. Pilates can help alleviate some of the discomforts of pregnancy if you take a few safety precautions.

Here are some do's and don'ts:

- Do ask your doctor for the current guidelines given by the American College of Obstetricians and Gynecologists (ACOG).

- Do modify all movements. The goal is to "maintain" abdominal strength and pelvic floor muscles, increase circulation, and control your emotions with your controlled breaths.

- Don't overheat your body. Exercise in an air-conditioned setting in the first trimester of pregnancy.

- Don't overstretch. You may find some of the exercises easier because the hormones flooding your body relax your ligaments and tendons. Resist the temptation to push yourself.

- Don't jerk your body into a move. Use slow and controlled movements only.

- Do consider hiring a personal trainer to work you out on the apparatus, especially as your belly gets bigger; it's easier than the Mat work.

- Do listen to your body.

In the Pursuit of Excellence

Winners don't distinguish themselves by physical strength alone. It's the combination of physical and mental stamina that makes a winner.

Enter Pilates! This ideal fitness regimen trains the brain and body simultaneously and harmoniously. The exercises train the body holistically by integrating mental tuning, visualization, and breath control, all while the muscles gain strength and length. By practicing the exercises, an athlete or fitness buff can achieve that edge, the fire in the belly radiating confidence. Pilates can help you maximize your athletic performance.

Sweat Isn't Enough

Today's athletes have enhanced their performances and have greater staying power. In fact, it's not uncommon to hear about athletes competing well into their 30s and early 40s. To train holistically, you must train the brain and body simultaneously and harmoniously.

How you sleep, eat, and take care of your mind are equally as important as the physical training you put your body through. Today's competitors have customized training programs that emphasize nutrition, stress management, and innovative and creative training methods that include mental preparation and physical performance strategies.

There is no mind/body separation. The mind tells the body what to do. The body, in return, does what it's told, whether you're aware of it or not. The exercises developed by Joseph Pilates are holistic because they integrate the mind and the body.

Every move starts in the brain. In a sense, Joseph trained as an elite athlete. Top competitive athletes, serious sports buffs, and anyone seeking a greater sense of well-being and deeper unity of body, mind, and spirit can benefit by adding his exercises and guiding principles to a training schedule. Here's why:

- You'll achieve a level of self-mastery by integrating your mind and your body.
- You'll develop your muscles more efficiently by cross-training.
- You'll reverse or prevent muscle imbalances, which can be caused by your specific sport. Developing the muscles uniformly is the foundation of every move developed by Joseph Pilates.
- You'll speed up recovery after training or a competition.
- You'll improve your concentration; it's this honed concentration that tells your body what to do.
- You'll develop breath control.
- You'll become more body-aware and disciplined.
- You'll improve your focus.
- You'll increase strength and flexibility in areas that were once weak.
- You'll better your "edge" by boosting your self-confidence.
- You can recondition your body.

- You can prevent injury by keeping your body flexible and evenly strong and balanced.

- You'll build core strength.

FIT FACT

There's not an athlete or sports buff alive who can't benefit from developing core strength, which is key to overall fitness. And most fitness experts agree that building a strong core is one of the best ways to prevent injury. Without core fitness, you'll get in shape to only a certain level, which means you'll compete only so well.

Training is divided into two categories: psychological and physical. The physical training is the grueling hours spent sweating it out. The psychological training, by contrast, is a combination of mental skills such as goal-setting, relaxation techniques, breath control, concentration, and visualization. These techniques can be useful to anyone who wants to develop a deeper mind/body/spirit union, not just athletes.

Pilates integrates the mind and body; it's a 90-year-old method that encourages physical and mental control as it strengthens the body and the mind simultaneously and harmoniously. Joseph Pilates said it best: "One of the major results of Contrology is gaining the mastery of your mind over the complete control of your body." Following his ideal fitness program better prepares you to achieve self-mastery for your sport!

With Pilates, you're accomplishing two goals: training your brain while strengthening your body, as well as improving your training and performance, no matter the sport.

Strength and Length

Strength in a muscle that's lengthened is the goal of most athletes. Let's take a classical ballet dancer. In most cases, she is extremely flexible, but she often lacks the strength in some movements. In contrast, a weight lifter probably has strength yet lacks the flexibility to move in a full range of movements. To a ballerina, lifting weights is out of the question for fear that her muscles will bulk up and she'll become muscle-bound. The weight lifter fears putting on a tutu.

You can have both—strength and length—without compromising strength or flexibility. Each exercise strengthens and stretches the muscles to keep them long, not shortened. In the end, length in a muscle means more strength. Why? Because you're developing more muscle fibers within the muscle itself. Therefore, you might even be stronger. Recent studies show that those who stretch after weight training can boost strength gains by as much as 20 percent! That means weight lifters don't have to don a tutu.

The research backing the benefits of flexibility is overwhelming. There's not a person alive who couldn't benefit from flexibility work. You'll increase your range of motion, reduce the muscle soreness associated with the postwork, and calm your nerves as well. And the payoff? You can lift more, your golf swing is more complete, your fastball is even faster, and your running stride is a little longer.

Pilates exercises counterbalance hard-core training in two ways: by lengthening the muscle after it's been shortened or loaded to the max, and by cutting down on muscle soreness after your workout. There might be a link between lack of flexibility and postwork-induced muscle damage, according to the *American Journal of Sports Medicine*.

FIT FACT

You can develop more muscle fibers within the muscle itself, meaning you might even get stronger by cross-training with Pilates. Recent studies show that those who stretch after weight training can boost their strength.

The more flexible you are, the less damage you'll have—although that's a hot topic for debate. Right now, there's not enough conclusive research to make that claim because injuries occur for a variety of reasons: lack of flexibility as well as muscle imbalances.

Muscle Imbalances

Think you're an in-shape athlete or sports buff? Look closely and take notes. Your muscles might have developed unevenly. Depending on the sport, some muscle groups are worked and loaded differently, while others are completely or partially ignored. Some overloading to the muscle groups can be caused by one-sided sports or by sports that don't completely strengthen certain muscle groups. Put another way, your muscles lack symmetry.

The Pilates exercises correct muscle imbalances, which is the foundation for every move developed by Joseph Pilates. Incorporating his work into your training schedule can bring balance and symmetry back to your body.

Preventing Injuries

Staying injury free should be your top priority as you refine your performance to attain elite status or your everyday fitness goals. Muscle imbalances, inflexibility, lack of self-mastery, plus a frazzled state of mind can all contribute to injury. Coping with an injury can set you back years or maybe even shatter your dreams to compete.

No sport gives your body everything; you must cross-train to fill in the missing ingredients, whether it's to keep you sane or to train muscles often neglected by your chosen sport. Cross-training means practicing sports and activities other than your sport to build overall fitness. Overall fitness usually cannot be achieved with just one single sport.

FIT FACT

Cross-training with the Pilates method can give you a break from your sport so you can build overall fitness. Overall fitness usually cannot be achieved with just one single sport, so cross-training is a must to prevent injury, burnout, and overtraining, whether it's mental or physical.

A New You

Clearly, you can benefit from Joseph Pilates' lifelong work, no matter your age or fitness level. The most wonderful thing about practicing the Pilates exercises, besides all the previously mentioned benefits, is that you finish with a pleasant feeling, as if you just rejuvenated your mind and your body.

Take a look again at the benefits of the Pilates method:

- Strengthens your mind and muscles
- Enhances your breathing
- Increases your flexibility
- Redefines your body
- Redistributes your weight
- Stretches your body
- Eases the stressful aspects of your life

- Boosts your energy

- Shrinks your waistline

- Perks up your bottom

- Cures most back pain

- Heightens your sex life

- Builds your self-esteem and self-confidence

- Shrinks your dimples—an anticellulite solution

- Develops both strength and length in each muscle

- Strengthens your core

The Pilates movement is not just exercise. Instead, it's the way to lifelong fitness and mindful health. It promotes physical harmony within each of your muscles with an invigorating mind workout. Your goal is to use your mind to engage your body to perform these movements correctly. You will then experience a whole new you.

The Least You Need to Know

- Pilates (*puh-LAH-teez*) engages you and leaves you refreshed and alert, with an enormous amount of self-confidence.

- Within every exercise, you work on gaining flexibility, strength, balance, and coordination.

- There are two ways to work your body: a group Mat class or an individually instructed program using the apparatus. You can do both.

- Pilates fulfills both psychological and physical training; it's a great way to cross-train for your own sport.

- Joseph Pilates' dream was for everyone to join the movement, from basic to advanced, from the injured to the super-fit, at any age and any level of ability.

Fix Your Frame

In This Chapter

- What your body's saying
- Getting a stronger, sexier back
- Getting rid of backaches and pains
- Striving for good posture

Call it grace, poise, self-confidence, or just plain sex appeal—some people have it, and others don't. Do you want a demeanor that makes others stop and stare?

"It" can be yours, effective immediately. Just follow the exercises developed by Joseph Pilates. They will lengthen your look and slim your midsection. The secret is a 90-year-old sequence of movements that works to gently elongate your back muscles, creating space between joints crunched by everyday life.

The Message in Your Body

What message do you want to give off about yourself when you enter a room? That you're strong? That you're confident? That you feel great about yourself?

Let's say you have a serious case of the slumps—your shoulders round forward. The message you're giving off, then, may be that you're painfully shy. That you have no confidence. That you feel insecure about your height.

Consciously or not, we send a message about our mental, physical, and emotional state by the way we stand, sit, and move. Good posture projects good health, vitality, and confidence, while slouching can imply weakness, feebleness, and self-doubt.

What's amazing is that this isn't a hot news flash. Most mothers, at some point, have instructed their children to sit up straight or pull back their shoulders. Current research suggests that people who have good posture not only are more attractive to anyone looking at them, but they also look taller and thinner. That's right—no longer will you have to diet yourself to starvation to look slim; just fix your frame.

ON THE MAT

Studies show that good posture is more attractive than supermodel svelteness. In fact, a 125-pound woman with excellent posture can be perceived as thinner than a 105-pound woman who is slumping, according to Don R. Osborn, an associate professor of psychology and sociology at Bellarmine College in Louisville, Kentucky. His research subjects consistently find women who stand up straight more attractive, regardless of their weight.

You'll feel better about yourself—and look healthier, thinner, and sexier—by improving your posture. You can also protect yourself from a lifetime of annoying aches and pains such as muscles spasms in the lower back, compressed nerves that intermingle with the working muscles, chronic neck pain, recurrent headaches, and decreased lung capacity. Good posture tames muscle strain and the aches and pains; helps you move with ease, grace, and efficiency; and gives your lungs more working room by increasing breathing capacity.

How does your posture measure up? Are you slumping, rounding your shoulders as if you're protecting yourself? Perhaps you're craning your head forward to see the computer screen. Or maybe you're a slave to fashion and prance around in the hottest stilettos (which, by the way, cause you to arch your lower back). Whatever the case, you're committing a combination of postural offenses.

Ask a close friend or spouse to take a picture of you. Don't pose. This shot needs to be as authentic as possible, so stand your usual way and strip down to your birthday suit (or your bathing suit, if you're too modest). Take several shots each of your front, side, and back views. After that, analyze your posture, starting from your head to your toes. Ask yourself these questions:

- Does my head hang forward?

- Are my shoulders rounded forward? Is one shoulder higher than the other? Are my shoulders tense, as if touching my ears?

- Does the upper part of my back hunch or round forward?

- Am I sticking out my chest, causing my shoulders to pull back? Are my shoulder blades sticking out?

- Do I have a potbelly—abdomen bulging forward—causing my lower back to arch?

- Am I locking my knees, causing me to arch the lower back? Do my knees roll inward?

- Are my ankles rolling inward as well, causing the arches in my feet to flatten and my knees to draw closer and closer?

- Are my feet splayed out, causing my knees to bow? In other words, am I bowlegged?

If you answered "yes" to any of these questions, Pilates may help. But first, let's get acquainted with your spine.

PILATES PRECAUTION

Attention, women! Women tend to suffer from more aches and pains than men. For example, we're often slaves to fashion; we love high heels. As a result, we tend to suffer from lower-back pain. Wearing stilettos throws the pelvis into a forward tilt so the lower back arches. Also, we tend to carry our children with one arm and hip on the same side of the body, which automatically raises the hip on one side and the shoulder as well. It's best to carry your baby in front, close to you, or to alternate your hips. Baby backpacks are great for newborns as well.

No More Pain in the Back

Poor posture stops here. The spine, sometimes called the vertebral column, consists of 24 interlocking bony blocks called vertebrae. Every vertebra stacks on top of the other, and these are supported by joints. The vertebrae provide back protection while the joints allow motion.

Then there are the body's shock absorbers, called discs. In between the vertebrae lie these circular, plump, jellylike discs that also allow movement. These discs cushion the vertebrae as you run, walk, and move. A finely balanced system of ligaments, cartilage, and muscles holds these vertebrae together and keeps the backbone from collapsing. Inside this structure is the spinal cord, a thick bundle of nerves. These nerves thread the spine's center to carry messages, including pain, throughout the body.

With perfect precision, these groups work together. If the spine is lined up correctly—*bone by bone*—with balanced muscle groups, back support can function without friction.

DEFINITION

Bone by bone means stacking your vertebra one at a time. This core concept is used in almost every exercise, so get used to peeling your spine up and down. Joseph Pilates used to say, "In coming up and going, roll your spine exactly like a wheel." Sometimes you'll read about "bone by bone," "vertebra by vertebra," "one vertebra at a time," or "peel your spine." It's all the same—move slowly and gradually.

To feel the bone-by-bone sensation, find a tennis ball and try this experiment. Sit in a chair with your knees slightly wider than your shoulders. Place the tennis ball underneath your chin. Begin by dropping your chin to your chest to roll down your spine, one vertebra a time. After your hands reach the floor, peel your spine up bone by bone until your vertebrae stack up—the tennis ball will drop at that point. As you roll up, feel your vertebrae stack up to lengthen your spine. Get to know this feeling because it's a core concept in Pilates—you'll stack your spine in almost every exercise you do.

Strain, pain, and injury can strike any of these groups at any time. Ligaments and tendons, for example, can be strained or ripped. The muscles that support this system can suffer a pull. The joints can suffer wear and tear and become arthritic. The discs, a delicate, finely balanced structure between the bony blocks of your spine, can rupture just by lifting too heavy of an object. If a discs bulges, it may compress the nerves, which can be terribly painful.

Still, if the natural curves of the spine become exaggerated, the bones press down incorrectly on one another, creating tension in some muscles while causing weakness in others. Put another way, some muscles constantly contract as the opposing muscles lose the ability to contract and weaken.

A classic example is having too much arch in your back, which is commonly referred to as "sway" back—but that's not an accurate characteristic of this condition. The abdominal muscles eventually weaken while the back muscles strengthen. One result: a bulging belly. Your abs go on strike, so your back muscles must work that much harder to support your frame. Muscles become unbalanced, and you end up with an aching lower back. If your muscles can't support the body correctly, then perfect posture crumbles.

FIT FACT

Eighty-five percent of Americans have suffered from lower-back pain at one time or another. Right now, eight million Americans have lower-back pain. In fact, back injuries are the most common on-the-job injury. And guess who's reaping the benefits? Drug companies. Nonprescription pain relievers are a billion-dollar industry.

How Are Your Curves?

Healthy, pain-free backs are made. As we age, a lifetime of poor body mechanics, on-the-job repetitive actions, and too much hustle and bustle catch up. Some muscles weaken, causing others to tighten. Every back can benefit from Pilates exercises because they restore strength; keep the spine flexible; and help maintain the natural curves of the neck, middle back, and lower back.

Take a look at the pictures of you your friend took earlier. Notice the natural curves in your spine. A healthy back has three natural curves and muscle groups that support the curves to help keep your back working fitly. An exaggeration of a curve, such as too much arch in the lower back, throws off the entire structure.

Take a look at your curves:

- The cervical vertebrae are the most movable and make up the first seven vertebrae of your upper back, starting at the base of your neck (called C1 to C7).

- The middle of your back, called the thoracic region, is the least movable and consists of 12 vertebrae (called T1 to T12).

- The lower back holds most of your body weight, and this is where the majority of back pain occurs. This is where you have your lumbar vertebrae, only five of them (called L1 to L5).

- Then there are the S1 to S5 vertebrae, the sacral vertebrae; these are fused into one bone. In most of the exercises, you'll be asked to anchor the sacrum to the mat. The sacrum is the top, flat bone of your butt.

- Finally, there are four coccygeal vertebrae, which are also fused into one bone; this is your tailbone.

The spine really adds up to 26 active vertebrae. The sacrum is one bone, and the coccygeal vertebrae make up the other immobile bone. The other 24 bony blocks make up your curves.

Got a Slumper, Here!

Are you a slumper? If so, you're particularly susceptible to annoying pangs of poor posture. Round your upper back forward, and your rib cage compresses downward to your hips. This decreases your breathing capacity. Plus, you've added an inch to your midriff, thus losing about 2 inches in height.

That slump causes your backbone to line up incorrectly. Common activities reinforce this exaggeration. Let's say you spend most of your day typing on a computer, craning your head forward while your shoulders round. As the bones in your back continuously stack up incorrectly, this causes friction, irritation, and eventually pain and wear and tear on the spine.

Compounding the problem is age. Did your grandmother shuffle around slumping her upper back? The *kyphosis* posture literally means an exaggerated curve in the thoracic spine. That's one reason why your grandma lost a few inches as she aged.

DEFINITION

Kyphosis posture means an exaggerated curve in the thoracic spine.

In addition to height shrinkage, slumping can have the following negative effects:

- It decreases your chest measurement.

- It causes your shoulders to round and narrow.

- It restricts your chest movement by pressing your rib cage down into your internal organs. Therefore, you won't be able to expand your lungs as much. The end result: shallow breathing, which reduces the oxygen flow to the body and brain, meaning less energy and vigor in your daily life.

- It creates a downward pressure, giving your heart, liver, and stomach less room to function.

- It may eventually create cervical compression and neck pain.

What's Up with Your Shoulders?

Got a hunch to go along with that slump? Chances are good that if you're walking around with a curve in your upper back, you're rounding your shoulders forward.

The shoulder contains many bones that assist in moving the arms. Even the slightest exaggeration can throw off how the left and right shoulders work. A misalignment that's too forward or back causes the delicate balance of the spine to get out of whack.

FIT FACT

Attention, men! If you can't live without your briefcase or laptop computer, you could create a height imbalance between your shoulders and hips by lugging them around day after day on the same shoulder. Try thinning out the contents. If you still can't live without it, alternate shoulders; otherwise, the muscles of the higher shoulder tighten and thicken while the other shoulder muscles weaken.

Try this: pretend you're Fonzie from *Happy Days*. Lift your thumbs as if you're a hitchhiker, but let your arms dangle by the side of your legs. Lift your thumbs up, pointing behind you to rotate your shoulders. Did you feel your chest open? How about a slight stretch across your chest? Your shoulder blades, the winged bones on your back, should have drawn slightly together.

Try this experiment again. This time, point your thumbs toward your thighs to make your shoulders round forward. Here's the muscle imbalance: your chest muscles shorten as the muscles in the back of your shoulder and between your shoulder blades lengthen, in which case you feel a constant tightness.

The point is, your shoulders should be in a neutral position. To do this, rotate your thumbs outward and gently bring your armpits to your hips. Now slightly draw your shoulder blades together to realign your shoulders. This way, your chest fully expands, giving your lungs more room to work. Put another way, you'll draw in no more shallow breaths; instead, you'll breathe more deeply. Translation: more energy. Of course, it starts with fixing the exaggerated curve in your upper back.

Is Your Head Straight?

If you're slumping and rounding your shoulders, check the position of your head. Does it hang forward? Lift your head as if a string were suspending it from the ceiling. The idea is to line up your head directly over your shoulders to stay aligned with your body's center of gravity. This relationship between your head, neck, and back keeps the rest of your body in line: head, neck, upper back, lower back, hips, knees, ankles, and feet.

Been bowling lately? A bowling ball weighs as much as your head, 10 to 14 pounds. The muscles in your neck and upper back work around the clock just to keep the weight of a bowling ball in place. That's why even the tiniest move forward causes these muscles to work even harder, which initiates the downward spiral of poor posture.

This extra weight disrupts your body's center of gravity, which can slightly change the curve from your cervical spine on down. Or maybe the slump caused you to hang your head forward. It doesn't matter which came first. This strain tightens the muscles in the back of your neck, which puts pressure on your joints and nerves that may result in chronic pain. A stiff neck, tingling or numbness in the arms and hands, and chronic tension headaches may be symptoms of poor posture. Look at the positions of your head, neck, and shoulders.

Too Much Arch in Your Back

Did you jerk up, jamming your shoulders back? So now your chest sticks out along with your rib cage, quite possibly causing your lower back to arch? Don't worry. It's a common response to go the other way. However, you're setting off a different set of problems.

The *lordosis* posture often creates a dull, aching lower back as a result of too much curve or arch in the lumbar area. Even worse, you're weakening your abdominal muscles. Look to see if your belly bulges out. Belly muscles weaken as the back muscles overstretch.

DEFINITION

The term **lordosis** means an exaggeration of the curvature to the lumbar region. Lower-back pain is most commonly caused by poor posture, especially in the lower lumbar region, not necessarily from "overdoing" it.

With that belly bulge, you're also getting these unfortunate side effects:

- Tight lower-back muscles that can compress the sciatic nerve, which causes a dull ache or stabbing pain radiating from your back to the tip of your big toe

- Knees that are usually in the locked position to support the overworked back

- Feet that are turned in so you're balancing the bulk of your body weight on your big toe and instep rather than your whole foot

- Tense, tight, often-lifted shoulders that weaken the upper-back muscles

Are you locking your knees? Does your belly bulge? Or do you suffer from a dull, aching back? If so, pay special attention to your lower back because these are all signs your bones aren't stacking correctly.

Try standing against a wall. Line up your heels and shoulders so you feel them touching the wall. How big is the arch between the wall and your back? Is there a lot of extra room? Only the palm of one hand should fit between the wall and your back.

Putting Your Pelvis in Neutral

Come on, admit it! You probably haven't given your posture much thought. I'm sure you, like so many of us, get caught up in the daily grind, sitting for many hours in an incorrect position without realizing that you're reshaping your bones and muscles. Maybe you lock your knees while tilting your head to hold the phone in place as you talk and talk.

Take a moment and visualize all the parts of your body. Get a mental picture of the position of your feet, legs, hips, and buttocks. Don't forget your stomach and how you're holding those muscles. Visualize your spine and back. Ultimately, you want to create length in your body, especially in your spine. You should be neither collapsing your shoulders too forward nor trying to stand up too straight, so your muscles and bones have a chance to *lengthen*.

DEFINITION

You'll read the word **lengthen** a lot—it means to grow yourself tall. This length comes from your spine, as if you're pulled up from the top of your head by a string. Grow upward to achieve this length, bone by bone.

Just by lengthening, you'll shrink your waistline, add a little height, add inches to your chest measurement, and provide more space for your working internal organs (such as your lungs), all while diminishing those annoying, nagging aches and pains that go hand in hand with poor posture.

To do this, you will learn how to move your pelvis to better get in touch with your abdominal muscles. Why? For three reasons:

- To lessen the arch in your lower back with hopes of reducing some of the pressure off your joints and nerves

- To lengthen your spine

- To get you to use your abdominal muscles rather than your already overworked back muscles

Try this: lie flat on your back and bend your knees. Feel the point or bony protrusions of your pelvis. These bony points are called the iliac crests. With the palm of your hand, rest your hand on this point so it's flat. Even if you're in a neutral pelvis position, you might have a slight arch in your lower back. You don't want too much of an arch, however.

Lift your pubic bone to the ceiling to flatten your lower back to the floor; no light should shine through. You're tilting your pelvis into what's commonly referred to as a pelvic tilt. On the other hand, if you were to drop your tailbone into the floor, then you're creating an arch, and light does shine through. This is commonly called an anterior tilt. Experiment here. Tilt your pelvis back and forth (which feels great) and return to a neutral position.

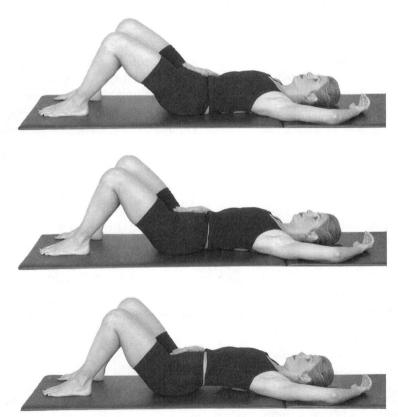

In a pelvic tilt (top), notice how your fingertips lift higher than the palm of your hand. When putting your pelvis in neutral (center), notice how your hand flattens as it sits on your hip bone with your pelvis in neutral. In an anterior tilt (bottom), notice how the palm of your hand lifts higher than your fingertips.

Supplying Spine Support

However poor your posture is, it had help. The muscles that support your spine gave up at some point. Well, not exactly—they got that way through habitual patterns. Just about every exercise developed by Joseph Pilates addresses the spine in three ways:

- To get you mentally working within your body so you can break old habits

- To strengthen and lengthen the muscles that support your spine evenly and uniformly

- To do every exercise in a biomechanically sound manner

By rebalancing the muscles that support your spine, plus mentally focusing on fixing your frame, you can reverse the downward spiral of aches and pains over time. The bony blocks eventually line up correctly, which will eliminate friction, reducing inflammation and chronic pain.

Balanced muscles, therefore, are the difference between a healthy back and an aching one. Each fiber runs in a different direction to support spinal movement and create support for your trunk. So let's meet the muscles that help support your spine:

- The *trapezius muscle*, or traps, runs from the base of your skull to the back part of your shoulders and then on down to the middle of your back to form a diamond shape. This muscle is often divided into the upper or lower trap. The upper trap lifts your head back and forth; this is also the muscle that tightens and tenses if you hang your head too far forward.

- The *rhomboids* are located in the center of your back. Try pressing your shoulder blades together; it's the rhomboids that protract them together.

- The biggest back muscle, the *latissimus dorsi*, wraps from your sacrum to your front ribs.

- The *serratus anterior* is located underneath your shoulders.

The Powerhouse

Don't let your stomach bulge; instead, use your *powerhouse!* The powerhouse links your abdominal muscles with your back muscles. For most of us, it's the most neglected part of our bodies.

To find your powerhouse, lie flat on your back. Place one hand on the bottom of your rib cage in front of your body and the other between your hips. Now inhale. As you exhale, notice how your belly button pulls back to the spine. That's your powerhouse pulling your navel to your spine.

Just about everything you do in life calls for your powerhouse. That's why most of the exercises in this book work your powerhouse. As you train, your abs, hips, and lower back turn into a strong center of support so you feel lifted, whether you're just sitting or walking.

Work the powerhouse, and you'll flatten your belly, get rid of love handles, and firm up your entire backside. The muscles work to form a girdle of support for the middle of your body and spine. Get to know the layers of abdominal muscles ("abs," for short). Each fiber runs in a different direction to provide a strong support system for your trunk.

Try this: in a kneeling position, press your fingers below your belly and cough. Did you feel the muscle contract? That muscle, the *transversus abdominis*, stabilizes your spine because it's the deepest of the abdominal muscles; it wraps, sort of like a corset, from the bottom of your rib cage in the front to the ribs in your back and holds your visceral organs in place.

DEFINITION

Joseph Pilates coined the term **powerhouse;** it's your girdle of strength. The powerhouse wraps around the middle part of your body; it expands from the bottom of your rib cage to the line across your hips and wraps around to your back. Your **transversus abdominis** will eliminate belly bulge. You'll work all your abdominal muscles evenly to create a firm, flat center; however, the focus is on the deepest of abdominal muscles, the transversus abdominis.

On top of the transversus is a set of crisscrossing muscles called the *obliques*. These muscles shape your waist and allow you to twist and bend sideways at your waist. If you point your fingers down toward your pelvis, you'll follow the pattern of your internal oblique muscles. Your external oblique muscles, on the other hand, run up the opposite way and lie on top of your internal obliques. Picture the letter X. Try bending and twisting at your waist to feel these muscles.

If you bend forward, you'll also feel the most superficial muscle, the *rectus abdominis*. It runs up and down the front of your body. Do a crunch, and you'll feel this muscle work.

By strengthening your core stabilizing muscles, you'll reap these rewards:

- Diminish upper- and lower-back pain

- Flatten your belly

- Shrink your waistline

- Lengthen your spine

- Fix your frame, for good!

Where's Your Body?

Clearly, posture matters. You should be aware of one thing, though: however poor your posture is, it might feel right to you. Start right now by thinking yourself taller. To do so, get in touch with how your body moves, and learn ways to control it. Quite frankly, that's how you'll get the most out of your workouts in the chapters to come, plus change your body.

Sure, every exercise works to correct posture, but it's not an overnight miracle. A certain amount of mental power will assist you. For example, you can prepare a mental checklist that looks similar to this one and practice standing tall:

- Stand with your feet hip-width apart to balance your weight evenly between your feet, knees, and hips. Keep your knees in a soft, unlocked position.

- Zip your abs by pulling your belly button to your spine. Remember the layers of abdominal muscles; it's the transversus abs that pull in your belly.

- Lift your rib cage slightly. Lengthen your rib cage away from your pelvis, for example, to reduce the pressure on your spine, which also shrinks your waistline. This length helps to correct a rounded upper back, giving your lungs more space so you can breathe more deeply. This also helps realign your head over your shoulders.

- Unround your shoulders by gently pulling them up to your ears, rolling them back, and then pressing your armpits to your hips to draw down your shoulders, away from your ears.

- Relax your arms so the palms of your hands face your thighs.

- Float your head up, as if a string is pulling it from the ceiling to lengthen your spine. You can gain as much as an inch in your height if you imagine this.

The plan is this: align! align! align! Align to train your body to feel what good posture is. Don't miss a day—align when you're sitting, standing, or driving. Tell your body what to do so your body will follow. It's your matter. Make it your mind, and eventually it will feel like it's your own.

The Least You Need to Know

- Good posture projects good health, vitality, and confidence, while slouching can imply weakness, feebleness, and self-doubt.
- Pilates exercises lengthen your look and slim your waistline.
- Your spine (your vertebral column) consists of 24 interlocking bony blocks that stack on top of each other.
- Your back has two functions: stability and mobility.
- Good posture relieves annoying aches and pains in your entire back—your waistline will shrink, your visceral organs will have more room to function better, and you'll breathe deeper.

Take Your Breath

In This Chapter

- Good health—just a breath away
- Getting the toxins out
- Tips for better breathing
- Frost a window with your breath

Breathing is a healthier way to wake up your body than, let's say, a triple venti cappuccino. Breathing jump-starts your heart, gets your blood flowing, and awakens every single cell in your body. This way, your body can carry away waste and even win the battle of fatigue. In minutes, a clear and focused mental state takes over where sluggishness once lingered.

Your breath is a life-enhancing basic function. For example, you can't heal yourself without proper breathing. Everything from fatigue to stress-related health conditions can be alleviated by better breathing habits. By following the exercises in this book, you'll feel the mind-breath connection Joseph Pilates purposefully planned to improve your state of mind and physical health. So let's take a deep breath.

With Every Breath You Take

For thousands of years, yogis (yoga masters) have claimed that your breathing possesses the key to a healthier life and clearer thinking. Westerners weren't so sure. Recently, however, a flood of medical discoveries have found that good breathing techniques can, in fact, enhance your overall health.

For example, you can use your breath to enhance your athletic performance and increase your stamina. Or you can slow down your breath to tame tension, relieve anxiety, and improve other stress-related health conditions such as heart disease.

If, for example, you slow down and deepen your breath, you can shift from a stress attack to a calmer mode. Deep, slow, rhythmic breaths can also slow your heart rate and reduce a skyrocketing blood pressure. Slow, gentle breaths bring a calmer emotional state, which can be a successful treatment for anxiety and stress-related heart disease.

Think about it. When you're anxious or angry, you often take gulped, hyperventilated breaths. This gasp of air reduces the amount of oxygen to your body, keeping you in a state of frenzy. If you slow down your breathing, however, you'll soon feel a whoosh of peacefulness overtake your body.

Use this same technique as a natural remedy for sleepless nights. Draw in as much air as possible, but this time, exhale in a controlled manner as you count to 8. While you do, set your mind free of the worries of the day that keep you awake at night.

If calmness isn't what you're after, you can use a percussive breath to increase your energy or to get the most out of life by enhancing your focus, concentration, and perhaps your memory. Coaches have used breathing techniques to help their athletes perform better, whether to calm their nerves or to pump them up for an athletic performance.

Did Joseph Pilates know this? You bet! You'll use your breath in a couple different ways while practicing Pilates: to purify your body of the waste that makes you tired and to charge your body with oxygen to awaken all your cells. That's why he brilliantly choreographed each breath to every one of his moves.

ON THE MAT

Joseph Pilates said, "Squeeze out the lungs as you would wring a wet towel dry. Soon the entire body is charged with fresh oxygen from toes to fingertips, just as the head of the steam in a boiler rushes to every radiator in the house." In plain English, squeeze out every ounce of air from your lungs so you can inhale as much as possible to charge your body with fresh oxygen—to give your body life! With every conscious breath, you'll feel healthier.

Breathe Like a Baby

Pay attention to how you breathe. Are you breathing into your belly as if you don't have a care in the world? Or is your breathing restricted by your chest? Restricted breathing could mean a few things. First, you've never been conscious of your breath. Second, you're emotionally blocked. Third, you never learned how to breathe correctly. If so, you're not alone.

Have you ever watched the belly of a sleeping baby? Her little tummy rises and falls effortlessly, as if she has no care in the world. That's one of the best examples of diaphragmatic breathing. Try it and see!

Unslump your spine, and take a deep breath. Breathe in through your nose and let it travel down the back of your neck and then to each bone of your spine, lengthening as it goes and goes. Drag this breath out for a count of 5. Try to make your belly rise. Could you do it? Not many can. Why? Because somewhere along the way you've forgotten how to breathe—and deprived yourself of the most precious gift: oxygen.

FIT FACT

The mind-breath connection was first discovered in India. When we're afraid, startled, or shocked, we hold our breath. The drama, then, stays with us long after the initial shock. By holding our breath, we lock the trauma in our bodies. Fear is said to be the root of many diseases. The Indian healing art of Ayurveda teaches you how to breathe properly, to unlock emotions that can eventually cure everything from depression to high blood pressure and stress-related diseases.

When you learn how to breathe in a full, relaxed way, you'll increase your oxygen levels, which can stimulate circulation and digestion. Deep breaths act like an internal massage for your organs—particularly your liver, abdominals, and heart—and helps them work more effectively.

Discover Your Basic Breath

Life begins with your first breath, and it ends with your last. You'll inhale about 100 million breaths before your last one. Your respiratory system includes your nose, mouth, windpipe, the muscles that support your diaphragm, and all parts of your lungs. Imagine what's happening in your body.

By definition, respiration is an event that exchanges oxygen and carbon dioxide between 60 trillion cells in your body. Breathing, however, is so much more:

- It carries nutrients to every part of your body. The cells within your body need oxygen to create energy and to carry out all their other duties.

- It increases your energy levels.

- It cleanses waste from your body. Toxic overload is one reason why you feel tired and sluggish.

- It calms you down.

- It connects you to your body.

Imagine two balloons. Picture them as they fill up with air; now let the air out. Your lungs basically work the same way. They fit snuggly within your rib cage in your chest cavity, filling up and deflating. As your lungs fill up and deflate, they act as an internal massage for your organs.

Between your ribs is a group of muscles, the internal and external intercostals. When you inhale, these muscles help pull your rib cage out, expanding your chest, while pulling in your rib cage or chest wall during the exhale.

Driving this action is your *diaphragm*. This thin, dome-shaped muscle sandwiched between the bottom of your lungs and the top of your abdomen acts like a pump. As you inhale, it relaxes and moves downward, creating a vacuum that sucks the air into your lungs. When you exhale, the diaphragm arches up into your chest to push out all the air from your lungs. Your ribs are going along for the ride, assisting in any way they can. To get more air, you need a good set of lungs; a strong, flexible diaphragm; in-shape and flexible rib muscles; and strong abdominal muscles.

DEFINITION

Think of the **diaphragm** as a pump, sort of like an accordion that you push in and out to generate music. When you draw air in, the diaphragm relaxes and moves down to create a vacuum, drawing air into your lungs. To get rid of the air, the diaphragm contracts and rises up to push air out of your lungs.

You can feel this up-and-down action best by putting your hands on your belly. Lie down, and when you inhale through your nose, try to make your belly rise. Then slowly let all the air out of your lungs through your mouth while watching your belly shrink to its normal size. Think back to the sleeping baby. Its little tummy grows bigger as it inhales, filling air into the entire lungs; the little tummy then returns to its resting size during the exhale. The baby doesn't fight the movement as her belly naturally rises and falls.

Let's say your belly isn't moving like a baby. Again, don't be surprised. For example, you may lose focus and let your mind wander, or perhaps you're used to breathing into your chest.

In that case, your diaphragm and intercostals aren't wholly operating, so your breathing is restricted. Why? Because stress, tension, and suppressed negative emotions can constrict your breathing as if it's held hostage by your emotions. You're guarding! Truthfully, though, it's easy to forget how to breathe if you're not aware of your breath in the first place. We all take breathing for granted.

Is this a problem? You bet. As it stands, up to a third of your lungs consists of "dead space"—no fresh air gets into these areas. This stale air zaps your energy levels. Fill your lungs with deep breaths, and you can exchange that dead air for fresher air more frequently.

ON THE MAT

Joseph says: "Lazy breathing converts the lungs, figuratively speaking, into a cemetery for the deposition of diseased, dying, and dead germs as well as supplying an ideal haven for the multiplication of other harmful germs."

Detoxify Your Body

Think of your lungs as organs of elimination that help purge toxins from your body. Your cells renew every minute, and old ones die. Toxins accumulate through wear and tear on your cells. In addition, you inhale, eat, and touch all kinds of toxins, and they, too, need purging. Toxins build up either internally or externally. Anything foreign to the body must be eliminated for optimal health.

Feeling sluggish? Unmotivated? Perhaps your zest for life has dwindled? These are all signs your body may be suffering from a toxic overload, whether emotional or physical. You can really help yourself by breathing deeply. A trip to the bathroom is another form of elimination. Blowing your nose is yet another. The largest detoxifying organ is your skin—break a sweat, and you're definitely detoxifying. Drinking lots of water can help purge toxins from your body, too. Think of detoxifying as the body's way of getting rid of anything it can't use.

Your goal, then, is to breathe deeply enough that all the cells in your body get enough oxygen. This can prevent toxic overload in the first place. But wait, let's back up. Your body produces energy in two different ways: aerobically and anaerobically. Surely you've heard of "aerobics"? By definition, *aerobic* metabolism means "with oxygen," while *anaerobic* means "without oxygen." Easy enough. Oxygen, and lots of it, we know enriches the body. Your cells thrive, and in turn, you feel energized and alive, and that's what your body prefers. But what if there's not enough oxygen?

DEFINITION

Aerobic means "with oxygen"; **anaerobic** means "without oxygen."

Two things happen. First, if the cells suffer from an oxygen debt, a buildup of carbon dioxide occurs. Second, for the cells to survive, they rely on the less-efficient anaerobic method. This backup system is not the way to go for long periods of time. If you were to sprint away from an out-of-control car or lift a heavy couch up several flights of stairs, an anaerobic state is the way to go. It's not ideal for long periods of time, however.

Besides being inefficient, anaerobic metabolism puts undue stress on your body. It produces a buildup of lactic acid and other waste by-products in the tissues. Muscles ache, and you feel fatigue. Have you ever pushed yourself to the point of exhaustion during a workout, chanting, "No pain, no gain"? How did you feel the next day or the day after that? Like someone took a baseball bat to your body? One of the contributors to postworkout soreness is lactic acid. When your body gets rid of it, you feel better.

But let's say you've lost some flexibility in your diaphragm and intercostal muscles, and both are not fully expanding. This happens if you're out of shape, when you age, when you feel stressed and hold tension, when you have tight abdominals, and when you're experiencing negative emotions. You're breathing into your chest. As a result, your labored and shallow breaths are not delivering enough oxygen to your body. You've just initiated a downward cycle to bad health: your body isn't effectively purging lactic acid, carbon dioxide, and other waste by-products of everyday living.

The good news is, you can reverse this downward spiral by avoiding as many toxins as you can. For example, avoid cigarette smoke and air pollution, get plenty of exercise, drink lots of water, find an outlet for stress, and practice your breaths to strengthen and increase the flexibility of your diaphragm and chest muscles.

Work on Your Stamina

Need some flex in your diaphragm? Or how about some stretch in your tight intercostals—both very healthy goals—to increase your lung capacity? What about building your stamina?

By definition, stamina, or endurance, is your capacity to perform longer without stopping to recuperate. Greater stamina, then, puts less stress on your body, and you might not suffer from postworkout soreness. You can achieve greater stamina with these breathing exercises.

No, you don't have to lace up your running shoes. Deep, controlled breaths combined with nonaerobic exercises also increase your stamina. At first, some exercises may be difficult, so you might need to rest before performing the next and the next. Use your breaths, however, to connect the movements so each exercise flows into the next.

PILATES PRECAUTION

Nearly 100 years ago, Joseph Pilates instinctively predicted that overdoing exercise would do more harm than good. His exact words were, "This infraction creates muscle fatigue—poison."

Eventually, your lung capacity increases because the two muscle types driving breathing—the diaphragm and intercostals—strengthen. Both become more efficient and elastic. Now you've got muscle endurance. You'll be able to repeat the exercises without resting as much between moves. Not only will you replace flabby muscles for toned ones, but you'll also build stamina. This flow reduces the time it'll take you to exercise. Good news, right?

Become a Better Breather

"Even if you follow no other instructions, learn to breathe correctly," Joseph Pilates said. Yet how do the exercises in this book help you to become a better breather?

- They help you become aware of your breath in the first place so you take the first step toward being a better breather.

- They help you strengthen your intercostal and diaphragm muscles, both of which are imperative to optimal breathing.

- They help you purify your body of poisons, including lactic acid and carbon dioxide.

- They help you get in touch with your emotions. Deep breathing can bring repressed emotions to the surface.

- They help you to heal your body and your mind by learning how to breathe deeply.

- They help you relieve stress. When you're going through a stressful event, carbon dioxide levels rise as oxygen levels fall because you're breathing shallowly.

In these exercises, we breathe a little differently. We're still breathing deeply—deeply enough to deliver large amounts of oxygen to the body. But the emphasis is on the exhale; it must be forceful enough to expel every ounce of breath from your lungs—to purify your body. Only then can you draw in a large amount of fresh air. You'll use your abdominal muscles to assist your breaths.

Wrap your hands around your rib cage, with your thumbs on your back ribs and your fingers on the front. Inhale to open your rib cage, filling the ribs in your back with your breath. At first, this concept may be a little tricky. You're not accustomed to breathing in your back—tight intercostal, diaphragm, and back muscles have restricted your breathing. Your abdominal muscles also are weak.

ON THE MAT

Joseph says, "Indefatigably and conscientiously practice breathing until the art of correct breathing becomes habitual, automatic, and subconscious, which accomplishment will result in the bloodstream receiving its full quota of oxygen and thus ward off undue fatigue."

Let's try breathing into your back: lie down on your back with your knees bent and your feet flat on the floor. Put your hands around your ribs.

Inhale fully enough to fill your lower lungs with enough air to expand the ribs in your back. Imagine an angel's wings expanding with each inhalation. Breathe along your spine. In other words, inhale through your nose, and let the air travel down your neck and spine, bone by bone, eventually to the ribs in your back. Even your shoulders flare out slightly.

Exhale through your mouth, relaxing your tongue and jaw as if you're frosting the window with your breath. Keep exhaling as you draw your belly button to your spine. Imagine your navel drawing up and under your rib cage.

Don't despair if you can't breathe into your back. This concept takes practice and some time to develop that kind of mental and muscle control. Your deep abdominal muscles, for example, have probably been neglected for a while; it's their strength that contributes to guiding your breath.

Practice breathing into your back so you can get this feeling before you start the exercises. Inhale for 5 counts, and exhale for 5 more.

Your breath protects you from injury. When you exhale forcibly, your deep abdominal muscles, the transversus and obliques, tighten around your spine to protect it, like a corset. If you're bulging your abs, your spine is unprotected. Picture your abdominals as a corset around your spine, getting tighter and tighter.

ON THE MAT

Joseph Pilates developed the breathometer, a small device that looks like a pinwheel connected to a straw. With the breathometer, he got his clients to breathe properly, which is essential to developing their potential lung capacity. If they could make the pinwheel spin, they could actually feel the power of their exhalation.

The Rules: Breathe Right!

Never hold your breath. Breathe in through your nose; exhale through your mouth, naturally, calmly, and deeply. As with all rules, there's always an exception. However, most of the exercises follow these instructions:

- Inhale on the point of effort.

- Exhale to a relaxing position.

- Exhale to squeeze your body tight or in a closed body position, pressing every ounce of air out of your lungs to protect your back.

- Exhale to flatten your belly as much as possible, with no belly bulging.

- Inhale as you straighten up.

- Inhale to initiate each twist.

- Breathe for the duration of the movement to reduce stress and strain.

- Don't hold your breath.

- Try pausing with your breath to let your insides expand.

- Breathe in through your nose, and exhale through your mouth as your jaw and tongue relax.

- As you blow out all the air from your body, pull your abs up under your ribs.

Avoid Running on Empty

Obviously, you're breathing enough air to get by; otherwise … well, you know. But are you getting enough fresh oxygen to reach your full potential? Now, that's a different story. The fact is, if you're not breathing deeply enough, your body can't do its job. You know, the stale air hangs around in the bottom of your lungs, poisoning your body.

As you age, the problem worsens. You can lose flexibility in your chest and lungs. Why? Poor posture! Now you're starting to see the brilliance of Joseph Pilates' lifelong work. If you don't work to correct poor alignment, breathing is restricted, whether you're young or old.

The key is to breathe naturally, calmly, and deeply. The inhalation is the inspiration for your movement and takes you through the point of effort, whereas the exhalation is the physical release.

Let It Flow

Joseph Pilates warned his students not to hold their breath while working out. Besides creating an oxygen debt, it stresses the body. In other words, you're wasting precious energy on muscles that don't need to be involved in the movement. A relaxed muscle tone makes more energy available for the move itself.

FIT FACT

Inhaling and exhaling 1 liter of oxygen burns 5 calories.

Vow to Get More Air

Short on air? If you've been breathing into your chest, then you're not getting enough air. Let's try to break you of that habit. From this day on, make a vow to get more air. Remember, without the help of your abs, your diaphragm won't get to pump away. Your diaphragm is responsible for 75 percent of the air you get.

Chest expansion can't deliver enough air, mainly because the middle and upper chest interferes with airflow. That puts the thoracic breather at an oxygen debt. You're working harder to breathe, which puts extra stress on your entire system. Your lungs work that much harder, as does your heart.

Again, look at your posture. Maybe you're rounding your upper back. If that's the case, work toward fixing your frame. Perhaps you're feeling emotionally blocked? If so, examine your lifestyle. Are you a type A personality? Is your life stressful? Do you suppress your feelings? Your joys? Your sadness? Years of tension can cause you to breathe into your chest. Enhancing your breathing capacity may help. You can also visit a breathing specialist, someone who specializes in emotional healing or bioenergenics, or see an Ayurvedic practitioner.

You're striving for freedom, emotional as well as physical. Get rid of the tension that holds you back from breathing fully and gain the good health you deserve.

FIT FACT

Stand up and yawn. That's right, a yawn is one kind of breathing technique. It's usually a result of a buildup of carbon dioxide in the blood. If this waste reaches a certain level, the yawn reflex is set off, releasing the stale air that sits deep in your lungs.

Trust Your Nose

Attention mouth-breathers: stop it! You're supposed to breathe through your nose; it's much healthier.

The nose heats the air you inhale and gets it ready for your body. And then there are the thousands of microscopic hairs inside your nose, called cilia. The waving motion of these hairs filters the air before you take it into your body. Any pollution, dirt, or otherwise no-good particles that aren't supposed to enter your body do not pass by the cilia. Your nose, then, is the first line of defense in the detoxification process. Nothing gets past it.

On a similar note, exhale through your mouth. Don't purse your lips together as if kissing someone. Instead, relax your tongue, lips, jaw, and face.

Tune Up Your Breath

Pilates teaches you breath awareness first. However, you may need to seek the help of a loved one or hire a breathing coach to help monitor your breathing patterns. Definitely pay close attention to your moods and how your body holds stress. For example, you may hold your breath during every minor crisis in your life and not know it.

Start a breathing diary. Think about your breaths at this very moment. Have you ever been in a situation that caused you to feel tightness in your chest? Write it down. How do you feel after an argument? For example, do you hyperventilate and gulp for air? In most cases, unpleasant events trigger breathing irregularities. If left unchecked, the cumulative effects can cause tight intercostal muscles or an inflexible diaphragm. The good news is, both are muscles, and you can lengthen and strengthen them. Are you getting your quota? Why not, then?

Monitor your breath while doing the exercises in this book. Look for instances in which you stick out your tongue or hold your breath, as you may have a natural tendency to do as you learn new movements.

Use your breath to help with a move. Exhale to release muscle tension, and relax the not-working muscles so you have more energy for the working ones. Stay calm, and breathe. Always remember the words of Joseph: "Even if you follow no other instructions, learn to breathe correctly!"

The Least You Need to Know

- Good breathing helps your performance, reduces stress, increases your stamina, and detoxifies your body.
- The key is to breathe naturally, calmly, and deeply.
- Good breathing may help defy many of today's most costly stress-related diseases such as heart disease, anxiety, and asthma.
- Full, deep breaths get rid of toxic wastes that make you tired.

(Re)Discover Your Perfect Body

In This Chapter

- Training tips
- How Pilates complements other fitness programs
- Revamping your metabolism
- Pilates training tips

One day you put on your favorite pair of jeans and think, *Whoa. What's going on here?* So you strip down and check yourself out in a full-length mirror. Hmmm. Your narrow hips don't look so narrow. You have a little extra bumper power around your back end. And your legs don't look as slender as they used to.

"That's it," you say with finality. You need an exercise program that will keep you motivated. No more erratic workouts, and you vow to curb your insatiable appetite. You need a fitness tune-up, Pilates style.

Spring to Life

Has your fitness motivation flatlined? Is your mind bored and your body even more unwilling, resisting change? Pilates helps you trim and tone your body, but it doesn't happen overnight. You'll have to make a commitment to working out, staying faithful to yourself. The ideal fitness plan won't change your body if you work out only once a month; you have to work at it! Making a wish list will help: "I wish I had buff buns." "I wish I didn't have to sweat during the workout." "I wish my arms didn't jiggle as much." Wishing won't change your body; commitment to the "ideal" fitness will.

The exercises in this book build up your body, not break it. Joseph Pilates said, "The workout leaves you as if you're springing out of the shower, not dead." Yes, you'll be physically challenged, but you probably won't be sore. Even if you feel a little frustrated, please don't give up!

The Art of Training

Even if you're an Olympic contender, don't be surprised if you can't roll your spine off the mat. At first glance, these movements seem easy, yet they're actually very complex. As Joseph Pilates put it, "Most professional athletes couldn't do their exercises properly when they started." That's why you have to concentrate while doing these exercises—it's the will of your mind that tells your body to do what you want it to do. So get ready to engage your mind to move your body. It's easy to do, if you remember the following guiding principles:

- Concentration
- Control
- Centering
- Flow
- Precision
- Breathing

These principles are interrelated with each move you make, giving your mind and body a makeover.

ON THE MAT

According to Joseph, "Ideally, our muscles should obey our will. Reasonably, our will should not be dominated by the reflex actions of our muscles."

Concentrate on Your Moves

Sure, Pilates tightens and tones your body, but it won't happen without the help of your brain. It's this fusion between your mind and your body that drives you to move, and that leads us to the first principle: concentration.

Concentrate on each move: the position of your head, the point in your toes, the arch or flatness in your back, the bend in your knees, and the rhythm of your breath. If you can *visualize* the exercises correctly, you will do them correctly.

> **DEFINITION**
>
> Today, many athletes use **visualization,** the act of strengthening their inner power so they can achieve the results they want. Train the brain, see your body moving how you want it to move, and your body will respond.

Control Is Crucial

If you don't move with control, you can injure yourself. Be sure carelessness doesn't carry over from your everyday life. Clear your head before you work out.

Quick, jerky moves don't deliver results any faster; they only lead to injury as the wrong muscles work. Be in control of your body, not at its mercy.

Discover Your Center

Have you ever studied yourself? Not just looked in the mirror to find a few flaws, but actually watched your body as it moved? Go on, check yourself out. Don't focus on the ripples; rather, watch your midsection. All motion starts here in your center, the powerhouse. Your center muscles support your spine, your internal organs, and your posture. By building a strong body foundation, you'll trim your waist, flatten your belly, improve your posture, and move with grace and ease.

Every time you work, the focus will be on building a strong center. The work will appear in many different forms, but you'll always be working it. Motion flows outward from your center; hence, the fourth principle is flowing movement.

Find Your Flow

Make the exercises flow. Movement should always initiate from your powerhouse with control and continuity. Never rush through any direction—no jerks!

Also, don't throw your body into the movement if you don't have the strength. You can modify all moves so you can progress safely to the next level without injury. Haphazard, jerky, and stiff movements are all no-nos.

Move with Precision

Picture the Olympic games. Think about the ice skater making three full turns in midair, or the high diver flipping through the air. These movements, no doubt, are complex, but the athletes make them look so easy, as if you, too, could do them.

Of course, we know these moves are executed with sheer precision and mind control. What's the difference between a perfect 10 and a very good 8? No doubt both routines are great, but it's the performer who flips with grace, ease, and perfect timing who earns the 10.

The Pilates moves call for the same type of precision. First, learn the steps to each exercise along with the breathing patterns. Don't forget about the guiding principles: concentrate on your body, do each move with control, initiate these moves from your center, establish a flow between steps, and follow through with precision. Fine-tune your moves; precision is the icing on the cake.

Precision transcends into your ordinary life. It affects how you walk into a room, how you sit, and how you carry yourself through life. Think through these principles every day so you can go through life a little more graceful and mentally balanced.

Build Your Breath

Finally, each step coordinates with your breath. Controlled breathing purifies your body, builds stamina, and reduces stress to your body when you're exercising. Even better, you'll find that your thoughts aren't as clouded. Pure, rich blood floods your organs, including your brain, with every breath you take. Deep breathing sends your body buzzing. Don't forget about the basic rules of breathing:

- Inhalation is the inspiration for your movement.

- Breathe into your back, to keep growing from within.

- Squeeze the corset a little tighter to get all the air out to make a pinwheel spin.

- Never hold your breath.

ON THE MAT

Joseph says, "As a heavy rainstorm freshens the water of a sluggish or stagnant stream and whips it into immediate action, so Contrology exercises purify the blood in the bloodstream and whip it into action with the result that the organs of the body, including the important sweat glands, receive the benefit of clean, fresh blood carried to them by the rejuvenated bloodstream."

Metabolism Makeover

Honor your muscles, find peace with your imperfections, and engage your mind to give your body the makeover it deserves. How? By increasing your muscle mass so your body burns more fat. That's what these exercises do—they increase your lean-muscle ratio, just like pumping iron does. However, instead of lifting weights, you'll lift, twist, stabilize, and control your body to get weight-training results without Herculean bulk.

Train Yourself to a Better Body

Maybe you didn't know this, but you've got the power to influence how your body burns calories—you can increase your lean muscle mass and reduce overall body fat. It's true—buff bodies burn more calories during the day than flabby bodies.

Your *metabolism* is how your body uses fats, carbohydrates, and proteins in the form of energy; it's how you burn calories. Whether you're doing absolutely nothing, running from soccer game to soccer game, or just breathing, your body uses calories.

DEFINITION

Metabolism is how your body burns calories. You can be doing absolutely nothing, and your body still burns calories. You can alter your metabolic rate by increasing your lean muscle mass and reducing your overall fat.

The concept is easy. Heat the body, and you'll burn more calories; cool your body, and you burn fewer calories. Guess what? Muscle needs more energy to function than fat; it requires more calories during the day, even if you're lounging on the sofa. The good news is that Pilates super-challenges your muscles. You can build lean muscle and reduce your overall fat, and in doing so, you'll burn more calories during the day to shape up your body.

Why not wake up a sluggish metabolism? Crawl out of bed and start exercising. During a 24-hour period, your metabolic cycle operates much like everything else in life; it speeds up during the day and slows down at night. You might feel sluggish when you wake up, but so does your metabolism. By noon, it's picking up speed; by dinnertime, it's peaking; and by bedtime, it's falling. So forgo that cup of java, and work out with Joe!

Eat Yourself Healthy

You can also give your metabolism a makeover by eating. Hold on—don't sprint for the refrigerator just yet. It's true, though. Eating raises your metabolism in a process called thermogenesis. Your body requires energy just to digest the food and absorb the nutrients from the foods you eat.

Your metabolism peaks at mealtime. It slowly progresses as the day continues, so let's keep your metabolism peaking all day, especially at the low points during its cycle, by grazing on six small meals a day. Even though this caloric burn is small in comparison to exercise, it adds up. But you can get double the caloric burn by exercising and eating a snack in the morning when your metabolism is still sleepy.

As another plus, you won't go hungry by healthy snacking. It's a better way to control your weight, especially if you have an erratic work schedule that forces you to skip meals. If you skip meals, you might have a tendency to play make-up-a-meal by eating everything in sight. You can end up eating a lot more calories this way than your body can use.

> **FIT FACT**
>
> Create a Picasso plate. Every time you eat, try to consume as many colors as possible, such as leafy greens, multicolor peppers, and a wide range of hues from berries. The more colors, the more disease-fighting protection you'll take in.

Don't forget to factor in healthful eating tricks. Eat mindfully. Rather than stuffing fast food down your throat, have a smoothie that combines two to three fruits to get five or more servings of energy-giving foods. You can also squeeze your own juice. For example, add a few carrots and Granny Smith apples, and you have a healthy pick-me-up. Now you're ready for Pilates.

Train Yourself Right—in Six Weeks

Ask yourself this: what do you want from Pilates? Chances are, you've started other fitness programs and dropped out because your goals or expectations weren't met. Or maybe you want to add a new dimension to your existing program. In any case, write down a list of wishes. Do you want a completely new look? Do you want to drop a few pounds? To get slim and sexy? To tighten and tone just a few jiggly areas? To be able to reach your toes? To fit into your favorite pair of Levis? To rid yourself of annoying aches and pains?

PILATES PRECAUTION

Pilates can be a wonderful way to get your body in shape and can work as a preventive program for many health ailments. However, it's imperative that you consult your physician, especially if you're pregnant, before starting any exercise program. Please get a checkup: blood work and a pressure reading, a cholesterol count, a stress test, and a flexibility test, just to name a few.

Let's make a plan of body attack. Decide on a time to exercise. Morning workouts tend to be easier to squeeze into a busy schedule. By getting it over first thing, you won't have to battle all the annoying interruptions of the day. What's more, that feel-good feeling stays with you long into the day. Yet deciding on the perfect time will clearly be a choice based on your personal best hours and whether you're a night or a morning person. Whatever the time, make a commitment and don't miss your workout.

Decide how long you want to exercise, keeping your goals in mind. If you want to slim down your body, exercise at least 45 minutes to an hour. If toning is your goal, exercise for 45 minutes. Be realistic. If you've never exercised before, take it slow, perhaps starting with 30 minutes; eventually you can progress to an hour workout. In addition, set a 6-week review to witness your transformation, no matter how slight.

Joseph says, "If you will faithfully perform your Contrology exercises regularly only four times a week for just three months, you will find your body development approaching the ideal, accompanied by renewed mental vigor and spiritual enhancement. Contrology is designed to give you suppleness, natural grace, and skill that will be unmistakably reflected in the way you walk, in the way you play, and in the way you work. You will develop muscular power with corresponding endurance, ability to perform arduous duties, to play strenuous games, to walk, run, or travel for long distances without undue body fatigue or mental strain."

Away with Aerobics? No Way!

Maybe you're a die-hard aerobics queen. You love to spin your heart out, or you enjoy the climb on the StairMaster. However, you're intrigued by the lure of the "ideal" fitness regimen. Do you have to give up your current exercise program? No way! Just add a weekly Pilates session.

The majority of my students already train in some other forms of fitness. Some spin; others take aerobics; some still lift weights. Besides the muscle challenge, they want variety in their fitness. That's a great idea because that's how you make a lifetime commitment—by mixing things up.

FIT FACT

Is once a week enough? Absolutely! Many of us do other forms of fitness and can squeeze in Pilates once a week. The strength, flexibility, coordination, balance work, plus breathing techniques will come in handy in life and in your own favorite fitness. You can also reap posture benefits. Obviously, the more you do, the more you'll get out of it—but some is better than nothing!

The Not-So-New Fitness

The question is, how will you ever know if your body is changing? Easy. Take some pictures of your posture as suggested in Chapter 2, or find some old photos of yourself. You'll be much more committed to achieving your goals if you actually see some improvement. And pictures never lie. Even if you don't like what you see, you have to have a starting place.

In addition, get hold of a tape measure and measure the circumference of your arms, waist, derriere, and legs. Jot down these numbers. Now jump up and down and take note of what wiggles. Your goal is to tighten anything that moves. Stay away from the scale.

After 6 weeks, you'll retest with hopes of attaining the first steps toward your fitness goals. For example, let's pretend your goal is to squeeze into a pair of pants, a pair you haven't worn in a while.

Don't deviate from your pledge to the ideal fitness. To reap the benefits, exercise four times a week for at least 45 minutes each day, and complete 6 weeks before looking at those pictures. "Practice faithfully; let nothing sway you," Joseph Pilates used to say.

Body Beautiful ... but Not in a Day!

You won't learn everything overnight. Notice that the exercises are divided per chapter. This is so you can safely progress to the complete workout. The introductory Mat exercises span a 6-week period, but you can advance when you feel comfortable. You do want to push yourself—after all, it's a workout.

Your goal is to learn all the introductory moves and breathing patterns, keeping in mind the six guiding principles at all times. After 6 weeks, reevaluate your progress. At that point, add a few of the advanced moves to your routine to keep your mind and muscles challenged.

Heed this warning, though: the best ways to learn the Mat exercises are through repetition and by layering as the weeks go on. Don't progress too quickly; otherwise, you might get frustrated if you can't do the movement.

Let's divide the weeks with respect to how you'll learn the exercises:

Weeks 1 and 2: During your beginner work, you'll focus on 10 moves, and each one can be modified. Let's face it, learning the moves along with the breathing patterns will be enough of an introduction. Try to complete at least 8 to 10 workouts with these moves before advancing to the next level.

Weeks 3 and 4: In the beginner-intermediate stage, you'll learn five new moves, plus a couple training tips to fine-tune your workout. Try to complete at least eight workouts with all the exercises up to this point.

Weeks 5 and 6: For your intermediate work, you'll learn seven new moves, plus training tips. These exercises complete the introductory work.

Your ultimate goal is to pay attention to each move and to execute each motion with every ounce of control and precision, coordinating each breath every time.

Joseph Pilates didn't just teach his method; he embodied healthy living. In his book, he writes about getting plenty of sunshine and fresh air, not overeating because it's dangerous to your health, getting a good night's sleep each night, and using a good, stiff brush to clean out the pores and remove dead skin because the pores of the skin must breathe. These were visionary claims 90 years ago, and now the science is here to prove him right. Don't you think he's a man worth following?

ON THE MAT

Joseph says, "Correctly executed and mastered to the point of subconscious reaction, these exercises will reflect grace and balance in your routine activities."

The Least You Need to Know

- The six guiding principles of Pilates are concentration, control, centering, flow, precision, and breathing.
- Your muscles should obey your will.
- You can revamp your metabolism by increasing your lean muscle mass and reducing your overall fat.
- Do the "ideal" fitness four times a week to make over your body.
- You don't have to give up your current fitness program—just make time for a Mat or a private session.

Show Me the Mat

There's a reason why Pilates is so fashionable. It works! In Part 2, you learn the core concepts, terminology, and Mat exercises. The exercises taught in this part are the same moves taught by Joseph Pilates. I introduce you to the exercises in the correct sequence so you can develop your body with muscle symmetry.

Befriend Your Body

In This Chapter

- Working from within
- The path of least resistance
- The Pilates concepts
- Mini-exercises to train your body

Go ahead and crunch your heart out, squat until you drop, and curl until you're jiggle free. No matter how hard you pump, looking your best comes from within. There's a certain "it" that brands a body beautiful—the way you hold yourself in any position.

Joseph Pilates understood the secret to attaining poise and grace, and now fitness experts agree. You need to work your body to achieve total balance and synergy among all your muscles. Don't despair. You can still tighten and tone the most eye-catching parts. However, the smaller, often forgotten muscles need a little attention, too—they perfect the way you look and move.

It's never too late to make weak muscles strong. The exercises in this book reveal muscles you may never have even known you possess. But before you start, you'll need to know how to stabilize your body against movement. Enter pre-Pilates! You'll practice several mini-exercises in this chapter that teach you how to get in proper position for the actual exercises that follow in later chapters.

So consider this chapter a warm-up. It's a way for you to get in touch with the new muscles you'll be working and to get to know your body a little better. In a sense, you'll befriend your body!

Body Wisdom

The goal of Pilates is to know your body. Your bones are covered in layers of muscles. Let's divide these layers into two groups: *stabilizing muscles* and *movement muscles.*

The inner, deep, stabilizing muscles hold your body in place, while the much larger superficial muscles move it. The essence of Joseph Pilates' work is to develop the muscles evenly so the muscles hidden below, behind, and between the more well-known muscles develop as well. In a sense, you're working from within because many of these muscles support your frame. The transversus abdominal, the deepest abdominis muscle, for example, provides a band of support around your midsection.

Movement muscles, on the other hand, are often superficial. You can feel them move your body. The abdominal muscle *rectus femoris,* for example, is probably the one you're most familiar with, especially if you've done a crunch or two. This ab muscle that lies close to the surface bends your body forward. It's also often strong, probably from overtraining.

DEFINITION

Stabilizing muscles are often deep muscles hidden between, under, and behind some of the more common muscles, while **movement muscles** tend to be superficial in nature. An example of a deep abdominal is the transversus abdominis; the rectus abdominal, on the other hand, is a movement muscle.

You can be fit but still be weak if you neglect these not-so-well-known muscle groups. If they get weak and give in to gravity, your whole body tends to sag, or the working muscles get stronger while the weak muscles get weaker. This imbalance can create poor posture and eventually can lead to a variety of aches and pains, initiating a vicious cycle.

If these muscles are weak from poor recruitment, the nerve impulses that control all muscles can't get through the muscle. Poor recruitment happens for two reasons: the muscles haven't been used enough, or pain occurs.

Let's say you're suffering from an aching lower-back pain. Most back pain, we know, is caused by poor posture. More than likely, you didn't work the muscles symmetrically in the first place. In any event, you've got pain, and you don't think it's a smart idea to work out with this pain.

Alleviating pain is the right thing to do, always! Yet question why you have pain. Ask yourself, *Is my aching back a result of me never working it or not working the muscles evenly?* This mental review is the first step. After you rule out anything serious, you can formulate a plan. If your back aches because of lack of muscle recruitment, you need to devise a plan that works the muscles of your spine and abdominals evenly. Otherwise, you'll continue to create imbalances as nerve impulses dwindle in certain sets of muscle groups. Put simply, the muscles waste away!

You know the saying, "Use it or lose it." It's never so true as for your muscles.

Training with Symmetry: Muscle Imbalances

Our bodies always take the path of least resistance, even if we're engaged in the most mundane task. Our bodies cheat, no matter what the task, because it's part of our subconscious.

Pretend you're a tad high-strung, with clenched, rounded shoulders that remain somewhere near your ears. This, we know, causes your chest muscles to weaken while your back muscles overstretch. However, your body doesn't suspect a thing; it prefers to function this way on a day-to-day basis, even during exercise. Not only will you have to recondition your body, but you'll have to do the same for your mind.

Your brain must be aware of bad body habits; only then can you alter your appearance. It's a two-step process, or else you're reinforcing bad body habits that show up later in life in the form of a twinge, a spasm, or an ache. Your body is a closed system, so if one part is out of alignment, the entire structure is altered. Misalignment has serious repercussions, and posture problems can affect internal organs' functions. So while clenched shoulders aren't pretty, your breathing also may be compromised in the process, and that will dull your vitality.

A symmetrically developed body is a beautiful one. Many bodies, however, lack symmetry. We're programmed to go for the burn. Many forms of fitness contribute to or promote imbalances by further weakening the stabilizing muscles. After all, we're working harder and doing faster movements to get that burn, instead of doing slow and controlled moves that develop muscle symmetry.

This imbalance leaves us aching, with our joints overstressed and our bodies vulnerable to injury. We've got tight and strong superficial muscles, while our very important stabilizers weaken as time goes on. Muscles work in groups, never alone, to move your body. One group contracts while the opposing group lengthens so your body can move. Some muscles overwork; others underwork. Muscles can become too tight or too loose, depending on how you use your body. We know this imbalance upsets your structure, and it's only a matter of time before you ache.

To correct the imbalance, you must do four things:

- Stretch the tight muscles, often the overworked muscles, which are usually the superficial ones.
- Strengthen the weak muscles, often the deep stabilizing muscles, including postural muscles.
- Correct any alignment problems.
- Develop core strength and stability.

That's the essence of Joseph Pilates' work—you'll flex and stretch within every exercise to restore symmetry back to your body. You don't have to figure out how because (thanks to Joseph) the exercises are perfectly arranged to work your muscles evenly. Just to give you an example of his brilliance, you'll "center" your body during every exercise by focusing on your abdominal muscles as a group to provide a stable base of support. Developing core strength is the very first step to attaining symmetry in your body.

For example, if you have too much arch in your lower back, your tendency will be to perform exercises with too much arch. So you haven't corrected the problem; you've only strengthened the muscle imbalances. If you don't correct the problem first, by centering, for example, you won't restore balance to your midsection, which could protect your lower back from injury in the long run.

You must have a certain amount of body wisdom to recondition your muscles, realign your body correctly, and change it for good. Sadly, we're not always aware of bad habits. So here's the first step: pay attention to your body. How does it move all day? Find habitual patterns such as cradling the phone receiver in the same ear as you talk, carrying your child with the same arm, or engaging in a sport that uses the same muscles.

Remember, you'll have to tell your body to move differently. Otherwise, it won't change.

ON THE MAT

Joseph says, "Contrology develops the body uniformly, corrects wrong posture, restores physical vitality, invigorates the mind, and elevates the spirit."

Your Cheating Body

Remember the first time you tried to ride a bike without training wheels? You might still have the scars! When was the last time you pedaled away? If you were to hop on a bike today, your knees would probably be spared the scrapes. Your muscles would pedal without you thinking about it; it's called muscle memory. You don't have to think about walking, after all. Your muscles do what they know best as a result of repeated moves for many hours. Your body automatically responds.

New tasks, however, require a certain amount of concentration. Your mind moves your body. Movements don't initiate in your bones, but deep inside an area of your brain called the cerebral cortex. This happens unconsciously in a matter of milliseconds. You see the movement and then your nervous system determines the best way to move your muscles.

Therefore, reeducating your body is not always an easy task. Many of the exercises you'll do require concentration; it's a mind challenge even for a skilled athlete. A marathon runner is often in great shape, with lean and strong thighs. His leg muscles can run for 26 miles, but if he were to attempt a Roll-Up, he might not be able to do it because he lacks core strength and flexibility.

It doesn't matter whether you're an athlete, a first-timer, or a client with poor posture—you'll need to concentrate, control, and focus on good positioning. If you don't set up your body correctly, your body cheats. Why would it work any harder than it has to?

Your muscles do the same thing. Stronger muscles, therefore, overcompensate for the weaker ones because it requires less effort. The marathon runner, for example, unconsciously depends on the strength of his strong thighs to get his body to do the Roll-Up. His muscles are asked to do something new, a move he doesn't have the strength for. So his muscles cheat, and his body follows along.

Eventually, your muscles will respond. Before long, you'll subconsciously know how to position the body. That way, you can build strength in areas that were once weak to have that "it" look. Remember, Pilates initiates in the brain!

Checking Out Your Form

Three main body parts—your neck, shoulders, and hips—are balanced over each other. Your center of gravity is behind your belly button.

You'll see it again, but start to think: neck, shoulders, and hips. Say it again! Neck! Shoulders! Hips! Run through this mental checklist before every exercise. Proper body position is vitally important to the integrity of the exercises. If you don't fire your muscles correctly, the moves are less effective. You also might not get the body you want.

While conditioning your body, you'll train your brain to work the same way every time. Start with your neck, your torso, your pelvis, each limb, and your feet. This firing pattern starts at your head and ends with your big toe.

PILATES PRECAUTION

When do you call it quits? Whenever you're tired, can't focus, or don't feel comfortable with the movement. If you can't keep good alignment while doing the exercise, the movements are ineffective. You don't have to complete the recommended reps—one perfectly executed move beats any number of sloppy ones.

Initiation: Learning the Concepts

You can learn all 500 exercises, but that doesn't mean you *know* Pilates. However, if you master the concepts, you'll reap these rewards:

- You'll continue to grow and not get bored.
- You'll strengthen and stretch all your muscles.
- You'll correct muscular imbalances.
- You'll fix your frame.
- You'll get the body you want (within reason, of course).
- You'll be able to apply what you've learned in Pilates to other areas of your life or fitness life.

If you memorize just the exercises, you'll get just that—exercises. In this case, you might get bored or unmotivated to work out if you can't continue to challenge yourself. This is true not only for Pilates but for any sport as well.

If you learn the philosophy, you can do any move anywhere and take what you've learned in Pilates and apply it to other areas of your life, especially other forms of fitness. You may want to train with a private instructor or attend Mat class, let's say, in Australia. In this case, the delivery may differ from coast to coast, depending on the instructor, but the core concepts are universal. Feel these core concepts in your body, and let them enhance your life, whether it's improving athletic performance or slimming your body.

You're about to learn a series of mini-exercises that teach core concepts. Each mini-exercise helps you get the most out of your workouts to come. This approach is gradual; it's a way to develop a solid foundation.

You can advance as you feel fit. Use your imagination and creativity to get the most out of exercises now or 10 years from now. You never know—you might be engaging in a Pilates class in Italy in the near future.

Learning the Lingo: Pre-Pilates

Pilates has a language all its own. Phrases such as "peel your spine off the mat," "bone by bone," "scoop, scoop, scoop," and "navel to your spine" conjure up all kinds of images. This is good because imagery helps. So when you read "stack your vertebrae," mentally picture your spine stacking one vertebra on top of the other. You'll read these phrases throughout the book. Have fun, and do exactly as it reads.

To do these exercises safely and correctly, you must learn how to stabilize your body against movement. This is an extremely important point: if you don't learn to stabilize your body before moving, you'll move incorrectly or move into your joint, which is typically weaker than your muscles.

So let's start by learning how to stabilize the main areas of your body with a few mini-exercises. Always work evenly in your trunk!

 PILATES PRECAUTION

Stabilizing your body before it moves is extremely important because it protects your body from injury and works your muscles more efficiently.

Transforming Your Transverse: Scoop

Think navel to spine! Imagine scooping your belly button in to make the distance between your stomach and your lower back smaller and smaller, as if your abdominal wall is right up against your spine, creating a flat back. You'll always initiate every exercise from your abdominals using this scooped or flat-back position.

Ever squeezed into a pair of jeans, lying on your bed and sucking in your stomach just to zip them up? This is the same contraction. Your lower abdominals pull your belly button to your spine so you can zip up your pants.

However, don't just suck in your gut; it's a less violent way to pull your belly button in and up into your rib cage. You might feel your spine lengthen and your back anchoring to the floor; these are good signs. You try it: take a deep breath. Slowly exhale as much air as possible out of your belly so your belly button pulls in as you zip up, up, and up!

By now, you're familiar with the superficial layers of the abdominal muscles: the rippled six-pack look of the rectus abdominis and the obliques. But the muscle you really want to get to know is the transversus abdominis, or the transverse. (In this book, the two terms are interchangeable.) This is your deepest abdominal muscle, and you'll use it in every exercise to develop core strength and to get what everyone desires—a flat, beautiful midriff.

FIT FACT

Every exercise begins by engaging your abdominals. The transverse abdominal muscle is vitally important to every exercise because you'll use it to develop core strength, slim your center, and protect your back. To get in touch with your deepest abdominal muscle, put your hands around your waist and cough. Notice how your abs get a little smaller with each cough; it's your transverse that pulls your belly button to your spine.

With a controlled, full exhale, you must get your abs closer and closer to your spine. Look for belly bulges on the exhale. That means you're not scooping enough to get your navel to your spine. In this case, you're not working the right muscles but building a belly bulge! By pulling your navel to your spine, you're ...

- Lengthening your spine.

- Stabilizing your center.

- Strengthening the often neglected powerhouse by putting symmetry back into your core.

- Getting rid of the belly bulge.

- Developing core strength.

Transform your transverse with the Pregnant Cat:

1. Get on your hands and knees, as if you're a pregnant cat.

2. Inhale and drop your litter of kittens to the floor—hence, bulging your belly.

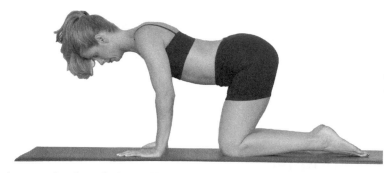

3. As you slowly exhale, pull your belly button in and up to your spine without arching your spine. Stay in neutral spine so your belly exhales in and up.

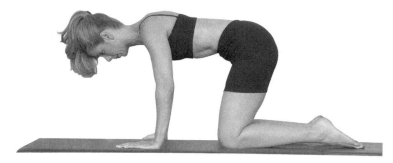

4. Repeat the exercise a few times until you can feel your transverse work.

Spine to Mat

Spine to Mat works together with "navel to spine." Remember, in and up! Whenever you read "spine to mat" or "anchor your spine," imagine your torso weighs 50 pounds. It's heavy, and it's anchored to the floor. There's no light between your back and the mat. Do this now: lie on the floor and try to feel every vertebra in your backbone and the back of your shoulders.

This "heavy" feeling protects your back from injury, plus it develops powerhouse strength. To get this feeling, lie on the floor on your back. Lift your legs in the air, with your toes reaching to the ceiling. You should feel every vertebra sink into the floor as your spine lengthens and anchors itself to the mat. That's the feeling you're going for, as if making an imprint of your spine in the sand. Now lower your legs slightly to challenge your back and abdominal muscles. Did your back arch? If so, you're probably not engaging your abs, or you might not have the strength yet.

ON THE MAT

Joseph Pilates called the center "a girdle of strength." All movements initiate from your center.

Peel Your Spine Off the Mat

If your spine is on the mat, you have to find a safe way to come up. Peel Your Spine Off the Mat curls your vertebrae one at a time off the mat, bone by bone. Think of peeling your spine up and down as a wheel turns.

Stacking your vertebrae, bone by bone, works the powerhouse, increases your spine's flexibility, and protects you from injury as you roll up and down. You must always protect your back—no jerky movements. From a Spine to Mat position, peel up, feeling each vertebra move bone by bone, called *spinal articulation.*

DEFINITION

Peeling your spine off the mat, or **spinal articulation,** protects your back as you roll up and down, increases the flexibility of your spine, and works the powerhouse.

"Imprint" your spine while peeling up and down, as if you're making a duplicate copy in the sand.

Practice Peel Your Spine Off the Mat with these steps:

1. Lie on your back with your knees bent and your feet flat on the mat. Your back is flat as you press your sacrum into the mat.

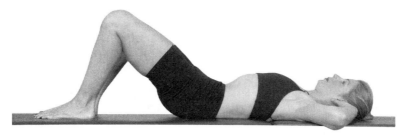

2. Focus on releasing the tension in your neck and shoulders. Let all your muscles along your spine relax as you sink into the mat, making a duplicate copy in the sand.

3. Inhale through your nose to feel your rib cage widen into your back.

4. As you exhale, sink your sacrum into the mat, starting to lift your pubic bone toward the ceiling. Feel each vertebra as it imprints into the sand.

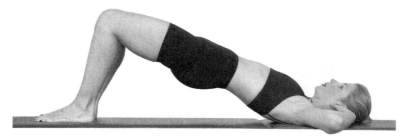

5. Inhale down bone by bone. Repeat three times.

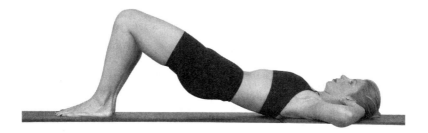

Chin to Your Chest

Your head is in line with your spine the whole time. Your spine starts between your ears and, because it's heavy, Chin to Your Chest is the safest position for your head, neck, and back. It works in line with gravity to hold your head in a safe position.

Try this: anchor the back of your head to the mat. Then place a tennis ball between your chin and your chest. Or if you don't have a tennis ball, take hold of your ears and lift your head out of your neck without dropping your chin to your chest. Do you feel how that position creates length in the back of your neck? This length stretches your neck muscles in your back, while strengthening your neck muscles in front and safely honoring the head, neck, and back alignment.

At first, most students can't hold up their heads, whether it's because of tight muscles, lack of abdominal strength, or pent-up tension. Don't strain to hold your head up; instead, put one hand behind your head for support or lower your head to the mat when it gets tired. As you develop neck strength, you'll hold Chin to Your Chest for longer periods of time. Let's try two easy mini-exercises.

Practice Chin to Your Chest using these steps:

1. Get into position, with your pelvis in neutral. Anchor the base of your skull into the mat, creating length in the back of your neck. If you're arching your neck, put a towel behind the base of your head to prevent you from arching your neck.

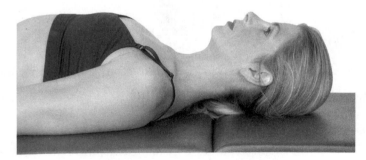

2. Lower and lift your chin with very subtle nods. Repeat five times.

3. Clasp your hands behind your head, and take a few normal breaths.

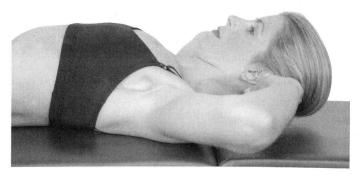

4. Inhale and lift your chin to your chest.

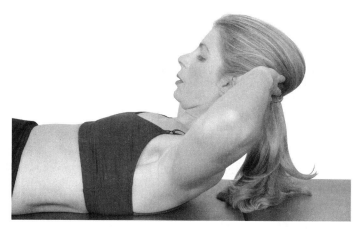

5. As you exhale, sink your breastbone into the mat, and relax your neck and jaw muscles—you should be able to talk in this position.

PILATES PRECAUTION

Don't jerk your chin to your chest. Create length in the back of your neck and then lift your chin to your chest. Your spine starts in your ears, so always work with your head in line with your spine. Most exercises initiate with chin to chest alignment.

Pits to Your Hips

Don't "hunch your shoulders," Joseph Pilates would say. That's not always easy, though. For one, that's where many of us hold our tension, in the upper back. Second, the back muscles that support the spine are often weak. And finally, these are some of the most overworked muscles in the body.

Give yourself a hug! Feel the winged bones that stick out of your back? Those are your shoulder blades, or scapula. Those bones, along with a few muscle groups, keep your spine erect and stabilize your shoulder girdle. Try this: bring your shoulder blades together. Do you feel your chest open as well?

Before any movement, it's important to stabilize your shoulder blades. In fact, these exercises strengthen the muscles that stabilize the scapula: the muscles between your shoulder blades, the rhomboids; the muscles that depress your shoulder blades, the trapezius; and the muscle that holds it in place, the *serratus anterior*.

> **DEFINITION**
>
> The **serratus anterior** is a broad, thin muscle that covers your lateral rib cage and connects to your shoulder blades. It holds your shoulder blades in place, which helps stabilize your shoulders.

If you press your shoulders back and then down, you'll feel the connection between these muscles. Scapula stabilization is vitally important to your posture and to protecting the joints in your shoulder girdle. Remember how your body lines up: neck, shoulders, and hips! Stabilize your neck, shoulders, and hips to align your body.

Stress throws off this connection, and because we're not always aware of pent-up tension, the problem compounds. After all, can you tell? Shoulders glued to the ears or one shoulder higher than the other are true signs that you need to relax. So relax and strive for Pits to Your Hips—shoulders down always!

> **FIT FACT**
>
> We overuse the muscles in the neck and shoulders. These muscles overtense and cannot rest or be released, so they remain active, in a constant state of contraction. Over a period of time, the muscles can't reach their normal length, and the movement becomes resisted, hence the "Quasimodo look."

Practice this, feeling your scapula draw down your back:

1. Go into a sitting position.

2. Clasp your hands behind your head, and draw your shoulders up to your ears.

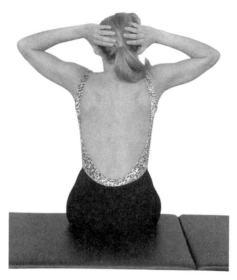

3. Draw your shoulder blades down your back, and feel the muscles that are preparing you for movement—remember, Pits to Your Hips!

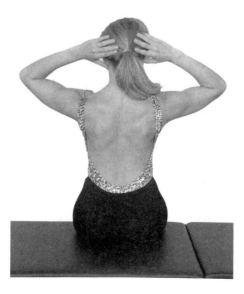

Pinch, Pinch, Pinch Your Butt Cheeks

Put a $1,000 bill between your butt cheeks, and squeeze—at least, imagine it. Buzzwords such as *squeeze*, *pinch*, and *tighten* should conjure up images of a tight bottom! But why? Of course, so you work all the right areas: your butt cheeks, the upper back of your inner thighs, and the ever-so-vital pelvic floor muscles that keep your internal organs and muscles from dropping out of your body. Imagine a hammock wrapping from the base of your pubic bone to your anus. Perhaps most importantly, hip stabilization works in conjunction with your belly muscles to develop core strength and stability.

Think about sipping a thick milk shake through a straw. As you suck harder and harder to bring up the thick ice-cream mixture, your facial cheeks pull in. The same thing is happening here except you're pinching in your butt cheeks. This contraction tightens and tones all the right places, so if you can't do this on your own, put a small ball between your thighs and squeeze it to tighten all those muscles. Keep it there until you can activate these muscles on your own.

Pinch, Lift, and Grow Tall

Try this: face a mirror. Sit up tall, and imagine that a string attached to the ceiling is lifting your head so you grow taller, bone by bone. Keep lifting so your rib cage separates from your hips, yet don't splay your ribs. This length must come from your spine as your head floats up, lifting every bone. Now pinch your butt cheeks so you grow even taller. That's Pinch, Lift, and Grow Tall!

ON THE MAT

You must learn to stabilize your trunk before any movement takes place. So the focus is on three centers of control: trunk stabilization—the deep abdominals (transversus and internal and external obliques); scapula stabilization—the midback muscles (lower trapezius, serratus anterior, and rhomboids); and hip stabilization—pull up through the inner thighs and pelvic floor muscles.

Joseph Pilates would say, "Sit up out of your hips." This position is a neutral pelvis, meaning no tilting the pelvis. You can really feel this connection if you sit directly on top of your *sitz* bones, or butt bones.

Here's how to Pinch, Lift, and Grow Tall:

1. To grow even taller, reach underneath and feel your butt bones.
2. Lift the flesh so you can sit directly on top of your sitz bones.

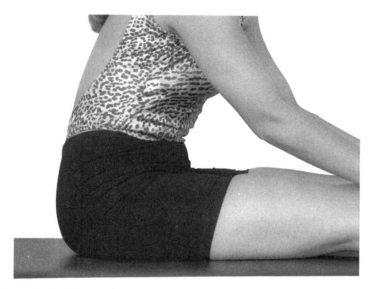

3. Now pinch, lift, and grow tall.

If you can't sit up out of your hips, keeping your pelvis in a neutral spine, put a small pad underneath your bottom. Tight hamstrings and overdeveloped hip flexors can interfere with this connection.

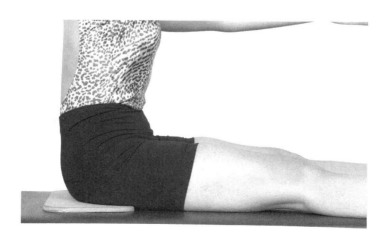

Just for Feet

Put work in your feet—take it out of your seat! In other words, don't point like a ballerina. Curling your toes over can throw your legs out of line with the rest of your body—or worse, it can cause muscle cramps in your feet. Instead, lengthen from the top of the big bone in your foot and then let your toes fall into a soft point.

If you're asked to flex your foot, lengthen your heel away from your face as your toes reach to your body. You'll feel a stretch in the back of your calves. But be careful—overflexing can cause your leg muscles to cramp, too.

Before You Go!

You can do these mini-exercises anytime. Trunk and midback stabilization, along with learning to lift through the back of your thighs and pinching your butt cheeks, are vitally important core concepts, not only for your safety but also for the development of your muscles. You're striving for symmetry.

These core concepts will stay with you no matter how you choose to train, with the mat or with the equipment. You've got to learn to stabilize your body for movement.

With that, extend it! Always think long from the powerhouse. You can reach a little farther, which is true not only for Pilates but as a fact of life—extend, extend, and extend!

The Least You Need to Know

- The three main body parts—neck, shoulders, and hips—are and should remain balanced over each other.
- A neutral pelvis balances your head, neck, and shoulders to line up your body.
- Legs and arms move from your core, your powerhouse.
- Stabilize your body against movement.
- If you memorize just the exercises, you'll get bored. If you learn the concepts, you'll grow—and that goes for any fitness program you choose.

Sculpt Yourself into Shape

In This Chapter

- The importance of body awareness
- Your mind's influence on your body, and vice versa
- Ten sculpting moves
- Understanding your scoop

Chances are, you've lifted hundreds of sets of dumbbells and worked your body into kick-butt shape. You might have fastened your bottom to a very uncomfortable bike seat to spin, and you might have found inner peace through yoga. Indeed, you might have sweated with the best of them. You're the boss of your body, and you're ready for the next challenge.

The movements featured in this chapter are the most effective way to introduce your body to the Mat workout. You'll use your body as resistance to lengthen your look, strengthen your muscles, and chisel your core. Along the way, you'll inspire yourself to do more, learn more, and be more as you beam with confidence—even in this first stage—as you conquer more.

A Perfect Ten

You'll cover a lot of ground in this chapter, so keep in mind a few things. These exercises are balanced and arranged to work your muscles symmetrically, thanks to Joseph Pilates. Do the exercises in order. In the first 2 weeks, do the following beginner movements.

- The Hundred
- Roll-Up
- Hamstring Circles
- Ankle Circles
- Leg Circles
- Rolling Like a Ball
- Single-Leg Stretch
- Double-Leg Stretch
- Spine Stretch
- The Saw
- Side-Kick Series (see Chapter 11 for directions)
- Seal

You're striving to maintain good alignment:

- No belly bulging—keep scooping, scooping, scooping.
- No strain in your neck.
- No jerky movements in your body.
- No movement in your trunk—keep yourself anchored to the mat.
- Take deep breaths to empty your lungs completely.
- No looking up at the ceiling—eyes on your belly the whole time.
- No hunching your shoulders—keep them back and down and reach long with your fingertips.

The message is clear: take it slow. Yes, it's these small, specific goals that make it easier for you to achieve your bigger goal. Think of these first 2 weeks as a beginner class. As the weeks continue, you'll progress to an intermediate class by adding more exercises, each with a different focus and degree of difficulty. But for now, stick to learning these exercises; it's the solid foundation for more stuff to come later.

Keep at it, and within a few weeks, you'll see a body line change that will not only make you feel good about what you've learned, but also dare you to show off your new bod!

Strike a Stance: The Pilates V

Strike a stance by gluing your heels together to make a small V, with your feet about three fingers apart. Turn your legs slightly out, beginning in the hip bone socket and continuing down the length of your legs to finish with your toes.

This V stabilizes your lower body, plus it works some of the most neglected muscles—the back of your upper inner thighs! Joseph Pilates always used to advise squeezing these forgotten muscles regularly.

Be careful—don't turn out from your knees. This could throw off the alignment of your knee, foot, and ankle. To get a better feel, turn your leg in a parallel position, with your knee facing the ceiling. Notice the straight alignment of your hip, knee, ankle, and foot? When you turn out, maintain this same integrity. Still, you shouldn't feel any stress in your knee or ankle joints. If you feel any pain, look at your turnout because it may be too much.

Strive to keep this small V position with your heels glued together during all the moves.

PILATES PRECAUTION

Don't turn out your feet too much or you'll put too much stress on your knee and ankle joints. It's a forced movement that should be reserved only for dancers. If you've had any problems with sciatica, check with your doctor before turning out your legs. More than likely, you shouldn't turn out your legs; work your legs in parallel instead.

Wake Up Your Body with the Hundred

Here's your warm-up, the Hundred. This move is a signature exercise developed by Joseph Pilates to warm up your body, preparing it for more to come. Regardless of the workout, the Hundred comes first to coordinate your breaths along with movement, increase circulation, and stabilize and warm up your core. Think of your lungs as a sponge—squeeze out the dirty water on the exhale so fresh water can enter.

You'll pump your arms about 6 to 8 inches, while inhaling for 5 counts and exhaling for 5 counts, adding up to 10 pumps of one complete breath. You'll pump for a grand total of 100 pumps, hence the name. While you pump, nothing moves except your arms.

If you don't have the core strength, your back may bounce off the floor as you pump. Think about the core concept: anchor your spine to the mat to stabilize your trunk.

Your neck may tire before your body does. This strain happens because of the combination of weak neck and abdominal muscles, along with overtensing the neck muscles in the front as you fight to hold up your head. You can put one hand behind your head to support or lower your head to the mat. You also can cut the pumps and breaths down to 50—quality versus quantity always. If you can't inhale for 5, reduce the breath counts. For example, start with 2 inhalations and exhale for 2, and progress to 3 and 3, and so on.

PILATES PRECAUTION

Attention all beginners! For your first several sessions, always remember to keep your limbs close to your center or bend your knees. Make no big movements and do fewer reps for quality over quantity. Don't forget, every exercise begins by engaging your abdominals.

Pump to the Hundred with this exercise:

1. Lie flat on your back with your arms by your sides, palms down.

2. Straighten your legs so your toes reach out to a 45-degree angle or are in line with your eyes. If you feel your back lifting from the mat, raise your legs to the ceiling to maintain an anchored spine.

3. Hover your hands about 8 inches off the mat. Keep them close to your body, palms down, stretching your fingertips long or pits to your hips.

4. Inhale and vigorously pump your arms up and down for 5 counts, as if your arms are pumping through Jell-O, resisting each pump.

5. Exhale the air as you scoop your navel in and up. Imagine a heavy ball in your belly button to help you feel your abs to your spine every time you exhale.

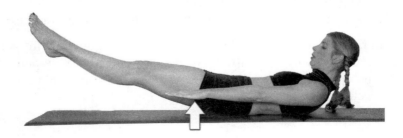

Modify the Hundred with this exercise:

1. Lie flat on your back, with your arms by your sides, palms down.

2. Pull one knee in to your chest, and pull in the other, keeping them close to your center. Lift your chin to your chest, and begin pumping your arms.

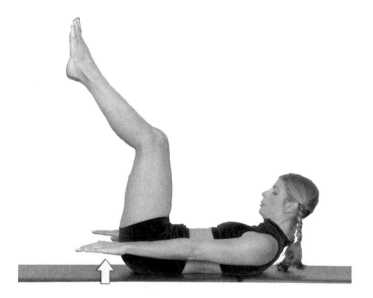

Roll-Up

The Roll-Up strengthens your powerhouse and keeps your spine flexible. A happy joint is a well-lubricated joint. The Roll-Up increases the *synovial fluids* throughout your spine as you roll up one vertebra at a time.

DEFINITION

Think of **synovial fluids** as WD-40 for your joints. When you move, especially in a slow, controlled manner, you're increasing synovial fluid production, whether it's in your spine, hip, or shoulder. This keeps your joints flexible, protects them from seizing up, and perhaps prevents one of today's most debilitating diseases—arthritis.

Remember peeling your spine off the mat in the imprinting mini-exercise? The same concept applies here. In the Roll-Up, peel your spine off the mat, scooping your navel to your spine the whole time. Imagine lifting a string of pearls one pearl at a time. That's how your spine will peel off the mat, bone by bone.

Watch out for clenched shoulders on rolldown; relax and let them hang. No jerks up and plops down—use powerhouse control as you curl up and down. If you find that you can't control the roll, try this: bend your knees so your hands can guide you up and down, or wrap a towel or Thera-Band around the front of your calves. Use the ends of the towel to guide you up and down.

Relax your quadriceps; instead work in your V and squeeze the backs of your inner thighs. You can imagine layers of Saran Wrap "wrapping" your hips together. This wrap will be used over and over again.

Roll up like a wheel in motion using these steps:

1. Lie flat on your back in the Pilates V, with your feet flexed and arms over your head in the frame of your body, dropping your rib cage, spine to the mat.

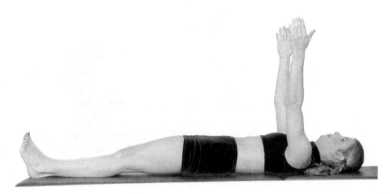

2. Inhale to lift your arms to the ceiling and bring your chin to your chest to initiate the Roll-Up. Press your heels away from your hips, and squeeze the backs of your upper thighs to control the Roll-Up. Fingertips reach long, while your ears remain between your upraised arms.

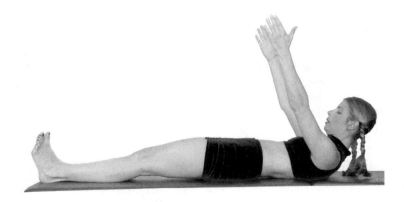

3. Exhale as your fingers reach long past your toes, and scoop even more.

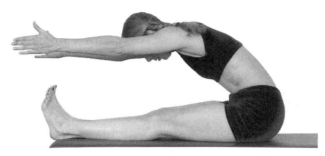

4. Inhale to scoop your abs and roll down to the middle of your back, pinching your butt cheeks. Press your heels away from your hips, and squeeze the backs of your upper thighs.

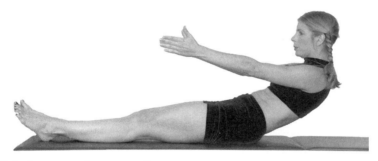

5. Exhale to continue to roll your spine down the mat, bone by bone. Repeat five times, as if you're a wheel in motion.

Flex and Stretch: Hamstring, Ankle, and Leg Circles

After the Roll-Up, stretch your hamstrings group to warm up your leg for the next exercise, Leg Circles.

Hamstring Circles

Your hamstrings are a group of muscles in the back of your leg that flex and bend your knee. The problem is, many of us either neglect this group or sit all day. As a result, the hamstrings shorten and tighten. Shortened, tight hamstrings can affect the position of the pelvis, which could eventually lead to poor posture.

Stretching your hamstrings can alleviate some of the tightness. As always, stay anchored so your sacrum touches the floor. Don't arch your neck or lift your head off the floor. Relax your shoulders. If you can't reach behind your leg or your calf, wrap a towel over the sole of your foot. Grab the ends of the towel so you can stretch your leg correctly. Don't grab behind your knee or lift your hip off the mat, thinking the stretch will increase.

To stretch your hamstrings, you have to square off your hips:

1. Inhale to prepare for the stretch.

2. Exhale to pull your belly in and up, and slowly pull your leg toward your face. Press your butt bones to the floor, and reach your heels out of your hips for control and to increase the stretch.

3. Pause. Release the stretch. Repeat three times, and then perform a series of Ankle Circles.

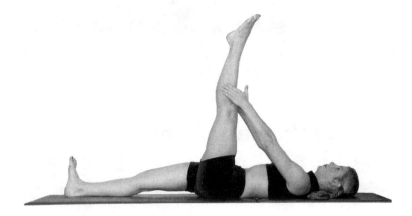

FIT FACT

If you allow your abdomen to bulge like a loaf of bread, you're no longer using your abdominal muscles correctly. Remember, transform your transverse. The abs are in and up under your rib cage—scoop, scoop, scoop.

Ankle Circles

Let's give your ankles some attention. Foot circles warm up your ankle joints, increase flexibility, and stretch some of your lower-leg muscles. Between lugging heavy bones and wearing tight, constricting shoes, your ankles never seem to get a break. After the Hamstring Stretch, circle your ankles. Roll outward five times, reverse the direction, and roll inward for five circles. Imagine this: you're splashing your feet in a pool of beach water and, as you slowly circle, the sand runs through your toes.

Don't forget about your often-neglected toes. Flex your foot by pushing your heel away from your face, and softly point energy out of your big toe. Flex and point three times.

Leg Circles

All this prep was to warm up your legs for Leg Circles. You'll circle your leg to challenge your trunk. Remember, movement of your limbs initiates from your core-trunk-torso! Leg Circles warm up your hips and joints, plus they tighten and tone areas that can't be hidden by a bathing suit: abs, thighs, and hips.

The hip joint is a ball-and-socket joint that has the ability to move in a wide range of movements. You can stir, kick, and circle your leg. Try this: bring your knee in to your chest. Gently press the bones of your hip until you feel the bone in its joint. If you can't feel this, stir your knee in tiny circles as if you're stirring a thick soup. Do you feel the head of the *femur*, your thigh bone, move inside its socket? As you circle your leg, this bone moves within the joint, reducing stress on the joint. You'll always work with the *bone in its joint*; you'll always stabilize your body before moving it.

DEFINITION

Bone in its joint means the joint is in its proper place. This proper joint alignment permits the limbs to move safely in a wide variety of movements without wear and tear on the joint. This particularly pertains to the ball-and-socket joints of the hips and shoulders. Remember, first you stabilize your body and then you move it!

You have two goals: stabilize your pelvis and prevent your hips from rocking side to side as your leg circles. To do this, press the palms of your hands, the back of your head, and the back of your arms into the mat to brace a very heavy torso at all times. Also, keep your circles small at first (as shown in the accompanying photos). Imagine a string looped around your big toe; it's pulling your toe to the ceiling so the uplifted leg is straight. If you can't straighten your uplifted leg, bend your knee softly.

Are you ready? It's time for Leg Circles!

1. Lie flat on your back, pressing the base of your head and the back of your arms into the mat, palms down.

2. Raise one leg up to the ceiling, slightly turning out from your hip, with your leg in line with your nose.

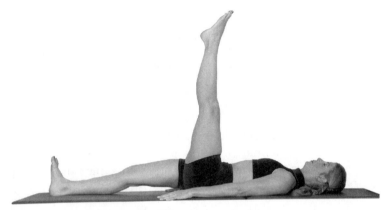

3. Inhale to lift your leg to your nose and take your leg across your body; your hips can lift slightly.

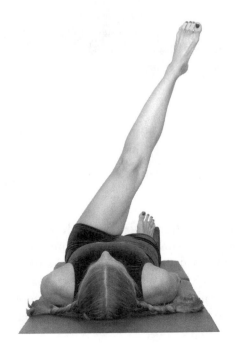

4. Exhale to take your leg down toward the mat, keeping your trunk stable and out to the side. Then inhale your leg up to your nose, stopping on a dime with a slight pause.

5. Repeat five circles, and then reverse. Repeat the whole sequence on the other leg: Hamstring, Ankle, and Leg Circles.

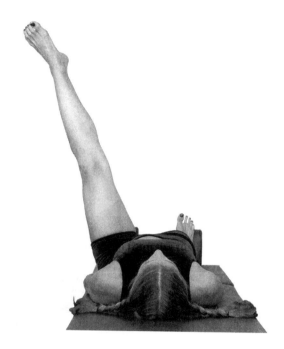

Rolling Like a Ball

Get ready for a spine treat! You're rolling to ease spinal tension, add balance work, and discover how to control your momentum in the roll itself. Momentum is typically a no-no, but in rolling, you'll use core concepts to control your momentum and increase the intensity: scoop your abs to your spine and pinch your butt cheeks together.

To get in position, sit at the edge of the mat. Slide your bottom to your heels. Place the palms of your hands behind your thighs, and practice scooping your navel to your spine. Try engaging your abs so much that your toes lift off the ground. Now actually lift up your toes so they hover about 2 or 3 inches off the ground. You may feel unstable here, but by deeply scooping, you can better control the wobble.

To roll with ease at first, you can open your knees slightly or touch your toes to the mat if you feel super wobbly. However, to progress, you need to focus on pinching your butt cheeks as well as scooping to roll without momentum. In the roll, your shoulders will have a tendency to creep toward your ears—don't let them hunch up. And here's the important part: keep your chin to your chest so you look at your belly button the whole time.

Do wobble-free rolls with these steps:

1. Wrap your right hand over your left ankle, while your left hand crosses your right wrist. Your heels stay close to your bottom.

2. Lower your head so your eyes are on your belly, chin to your chest. Your head will never touch the mat. Don't scrunch your spine; it's a lift up and over!

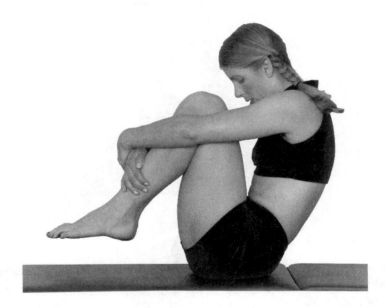

3. Inhale as you roll back, pinch your butt cheeks, scoop your belly, and lift your tailbone to the ceiling. Stay tight.

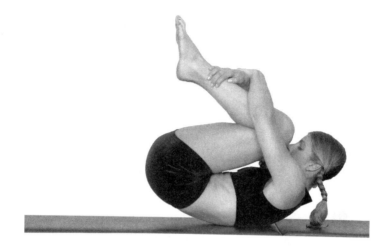

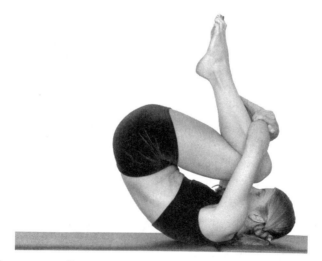

4. Exhale as you roll up, and scoop your belly to protect your lower back—no belly bulge.

5. Repeat 8 to 10 times, keeping the motion going.

ON THE MAT

Rolling Like a Ball is among Pilates' brilliant moves. The "rolling" is a good example of driving out the impurities. As you roll and unroll your spine—vertebra by vertebra—you're cleansing your lungs.

Single- and Double-Leg Stretch

The warm-up is over! You're now increasing the intensity, starting with the Single-Leg Stretch, which uses 100 percent pure abs. This stretch initiates a series of ab exercises known as the "fives." You'll do the "twos," however. Like the Hundred, these exercises coordinate breath and ab work as you move your limbs and stabilize your torso. They require a great deal of coordination and concentration.

Single-Leg Stretch

So where's the stretch? Imagine your leg stretching for miles and miles—1, 2, 3 miles long as your big toe lengthens away from your hips. Your toe is in line with your nose; pinch your butt cheeks, and use those thighs! Your neck may tire first, so be sure your chin is on your chest and your eyes look at your navel the whole time. Lower your head if you feel any neck strain. Don't stop the exercise, though. Lift your head into position after a little rest.

Start your intense ab work with the Single-Leg Stretch:

1. Anchor your spine to the mat. Bring your knees in to your chest. At the same time, stretch your left leg so your toe is in line with your nose. Place your right hand on the outside of your right ankle or near it, while your left hand rests on the inside of your right knee, your elbows wide. This hand position keeps your knee aligned with your ankle, knee, and hip.

2. Lift your chin to your chest, and stretch your left leg long, softly pointing your toes, a couple inches off the mat or higher, depending on where you can anchor your spine. Inhale gradually for two leg stretches.

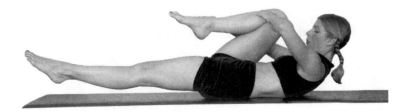

3. Exhale as you switch your legs and lengthen away from your hips for two stretches. Blow all the air out of your lungs to flatten your belly. Pull your left leg in to your chest as your right foot lengthens long. Keep your leg high to secure your back to the mat, if needed. As your core strength improves, you'll skim the mat with your toes.

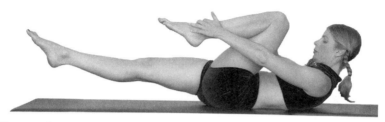

4. Repeat four to eight stretches, with eight stretches per leg.

Double-Leg Stretch

Rest for a minute and then continue this ab series with the Double-Leg Stretch. As your core strength develops, you won't need to rest. In addition to developing your core, you're testing your coordination and endurance.

Up the ab work with these steps:

1. Recheck your body. If you need to anchor your spine, do so.

2. Draw your knees in to your chest. Place your hands on your shins. Keep your chin on your chest, and scoop your belly.

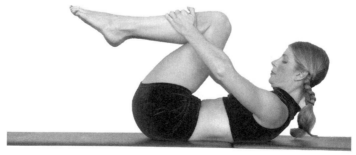

3. Press your legs, if you can, in to your chest to blow out all the air. Inhale to extend all four limbs to the ceiling—or out to a 45-degree angle, depending on your ability to anchor your spine. At no time should you arch your back; keep a firm and stable trunk.

4. Exhale and gracefully circle your arms, with your hands toward the ceiling and then behind your head, stretching your fingers long over your head. At the same time, reach your toes long. Your arms move a second or two before your legs. Your legs follow your arms in to your chest to the start position. Your trunk never moves!

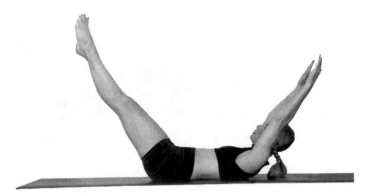

5. Repeat five smooth, flowing stretches.

FIT FACT

If you find that your belly muscles are outlasting your neck, you have a few options. You could put your hands behind your head to support your neck, or you could lower your head to the floor. If you still feel the exercise is too stressful, use a small pillow to support your head and neck.

Spine Stretch

Finally, a stretch. You've earned it after all that hard abdominal work. Let's stretch your spine and hamstrings, plus reinforce your commitment to stacking your spine bone by bone. During this stretch, be sure you empty your lungs and inhale. Remember, your lungs are like a sponge!

1. Sit on the mat with your legs spread a little more than shoulder width.

2. Anchor your butt bones to the mat. Pinch, lift, and grow tall. Remain committed to your scoop, in and up.

3. Flex your toes so you feel a stretch in your hamstrings, but don't lock your knees. Inhale into your back.

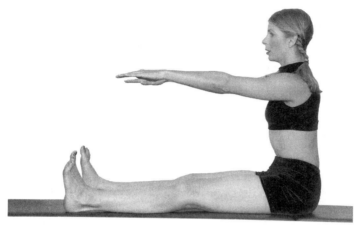

4. Exhale and lower your chin to your chest, curling the top of your head toward the floor, scooping the whole time. Aim your nose toward your tailbone.

5. At the same time, stretch your fingertips, extending past an imaginary line running between your feet. Even though your arms are stretching forward, keep scooping your navel to your spine. When you've stretched to your limits, pause.

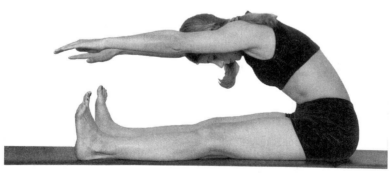

6. Inhale into your back to restack your spine while pressing the back of your legs into the mat to secure your bottom.

7. Repeat five times, even though you'll be tempted to do more.

The Saw

Joseph Pilates said, "Wring out the lungs like a dish towel." In the Saw, you'll twist your torso to wring out your lungs of all their impurities. It's a waist-trimming exercise to strengthen your obliques and also stretch your hamstrings.

Imagine your belly button lifting and then twisting your torso as you reach for your little toe to saw it off. Focus on the up and over.

Learn the Saw using these steps:

1. Sit on the mat with your legs straight out in front of you, a little wider than shoulder width.

2. Anchor your heels and butt bones to the mat, and scoop. Raise your arms straight out at your sides, and pull them apart, palms down and reaching your fingertips long. Inhale to grow tall, lift your ribs off your pelvis, and initiate the twist.

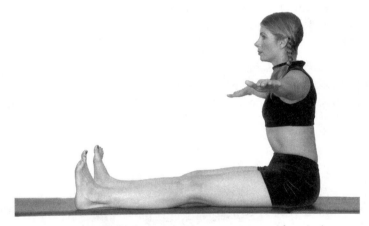

3. Exhale deeper into the twist. Imagine your navel twisting your torso as your right hand reaches past your left foot, as if sawing off your pinky toe. Your ear listens to your knee as you look behind to twist a little farther, each time exhaling every ounce of air out of your lungs; it's not a bounce.

4. To get the most from this stretch, reach your left hand behind you, turning your palm up. Inhale and return to the starting position even taller—pinch, lift, and grow! Exhale to twist the other way.

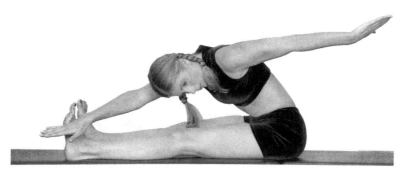

5. Repeat three or four sets.

FIT FACT

To sit up out of your hips, visualize your head floating up, up, up to the clouds. Use your inner thighs, lower tush, and belly to help create length all the way up your spine. If you're collapsing in your hips, meaning you can't sit up out of your hips, then place a small pad under your butt.

Seal

Bark like a seal, and clap your heels together. Sound ridiculous? That's how your Pilates Mat class ends. What's the point? It's fun, relieves tension in your spine, and works on balance and control. This clap comes from your hips, not your feet, to make the powerhouse work. At first, clap in front. As you advance, you can clap in both directions, in front and overhead.

Here are the steps you'll use:

1. Wrap your arms under your legs, reaching under your knees, outside your ankles, to grab your feet—about 1 inch from the floor.

2. Heels together, clap your heels and bark like a seal. Just warming up! Scoop and look at your belly the whole time.

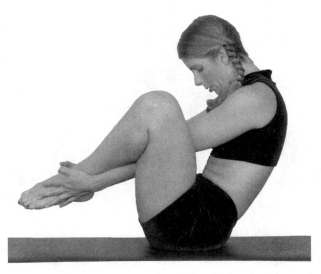

3. Inhale to roll back, lifting your butt cheeks in the air—pinching the entire time—until your weight shifts to your shoulder blades. For the advanced, clap while balancing on your shoulder blades 1 inch from the floor.

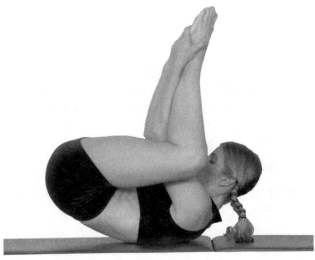

4. Exhale to roll up, scooping your belly, focusing on your navel. Balance and clap your heels together. Repeat 8 to 10 times.

Wrapping It Up

The message is clear: Joseph Pilates rules. Even in the earlier stages, you can develop strength and flexibility in each muscle, work on coordination, and de-wobble your body. These exercises were perfectly arranged to give you a total body workout.

Try to commit these exercises to memory. As you see, the core concepts are used in every move, no matter what. Be kind to yourself if you feel a little uncoordinated or wobbly. The movements take time to penetrate your mind and body.

You won't build strength overnight, so don't rush the movement or learning—remember, quality over quantity. After all, you have a lifetime to enjoy the range of exercises and benefits. Relax, stick with it, and scoop, scoop, scoop!

The Least You Need to Know

- To strike a Pilates V, glue your heels and thighs together, with your toes about 3 inches apart.
- Do the exercises in order because that's how Joseph Pilates arranged them to work the muscles symmetrically.
- Layer the moves to build a solid foundation; it's these small, specific goals that make it easy to achieve the bigger goal.

Get the Man-Made Mat Body

In This Chapter

- Never do a crunch again!
- Recommit to your scoop
- Learn the principles of overload
- Strong and long

Great bodies are made, not born! It's the subtle curves of the thigh, the rippling of the abs, the lift in the derriere, and the sculpted arms that make a body good-looking.

So how can you get a good-looking body? You have to create it yourself, and there's no way around it. For a sleek, strong, well-toned body, you have to move your body a new way and add resistance to your workout. You must challenge your muscles even if you're devoted to your workout.

Your goal is to activate more muscle fibers: go slow, hold your body a little longer, squeeze each muscle, and challenge your muscles with a little extra body weight. The results? A man-made bod!

Busting Your Gut

Crunches didn't work for you? You're not alone. Millions have crunched their bellies into a big fat bulge. So why did we do it? Perhaps it was to get rid of our back pain. We've heard that strong abs can lessen the workload of our back muscles, which is true. Or maybe it was pure vanity; we wanted that rippled six-pack look. Whatever the reason, we crunched our heart out for nothing—a bulging potbelly. How discouraging!

Traditionally, there's the crunch or a sit-up. Both abdominal exercises strengthen muscles but not always your abs. Actually, instead of flattening your midsection, you've probably given your hip flexors a workout. The major hip flexor muscle, *illiopsoas* (or psoas for short), starts in the crease of your upper thigh and wraps through the pelvis to attach to the lumbar vertebrae—it lifts your knee to your chest.

When you crunch, or do a sit-up, the psoas muscle responds probably more than your abs. Why? Because this muscle is often tight from overuse and strong from being overdeveloped, which can cause lower-back pain in the end.

FIT FACT

If you're not positioning your body correctly when performing a crunch or sit-up, you're creating a monster bulge in your belly rather than the sleek and slender abs you so deserve.

Securing Your Scoop

If you jerk up when doing a sit-up or crunch, either your psoas is tight from being overworked or you don't have the ab strength—or perhaps a combination of both. Neither scenario is good because you'll probably feel this "spring" in your back. Let's say you have a combination of strong hip flexors and weak abs, yet you're determined to do a sit-up. You'll get up; however, your tight, shortened hip flexor responds by pulling your lumbar vertebrae into play. When this happens, your lower back arches, which also naturally slightly bulges or distends your belly. Consequently, you'll feel a tug in your lower back.

If you continue to sit up or crunch without securing your scoop, you'll end up with a combination of weak abs, even tighter psoas, and a bigger muscle monster bulge. Try it for yourself.

To sit up, crunch, or roll your spine into an upright position safely, you need less hip flexors and more abdominal strength. To do this, you must maintain a neutral pelvis and simply scoop! That's one reason why the Roll-Up is such an effective midsection reducer and core strengthener.

First, you anchor your spine and scoop your belly button before any movement; it's called centering. Not only does this position flatten your belly, but it also protects your back. Second, you're told to keep your head in line with your spine the whole time. Finally, you peel your spine off the mat, bone by bone. The movement, then, becomes a slow and controlled one rather than a series of jerk-ups.

The Strong and Long

Elongation during the entire movement, through full range of motion, is a must to create a long and strong body. We've been conditioned to believe it takes mega-reps with lots of weight to build muscle strength. That's not always the case, though. In fact, if the muscle tires, it works in a contracted or shortened length. Muscles can work easier in a contracted state, so what you're really developing is strength and bulge.

Your muscles contract three ways: *isometrically*, *concentrically*, and *eccentrically*. If you work without balance between the muscle groups, imbalance happens. Concentric contraction shortens the muscles as it contracts; for example, a biceps curl shortens the biceps muscle. If you reverse the direction, then you're lengthening the muscle, which is an eccentric contraction. Isometric contractions hold the muscle in place to create a static muscle contraction.

DEFINITION

A **concentric contraction** shortens the muscle, while an **eccentric contraction** lengthens the muscle. For example, if you do a bicep curl, you're shortening the muscle. Reverse the curl, and now you're lengthening the muscle. During **isometric contractions,** the muscle doesn't move.

If you're not lengthening the muscle by working in a full range of motion, then you're shortening it. Not to pick on the crunch, but this abdominal exercise provides the perfect example of how you shorten a muscle: the emphasis is to bend forward—crunch, crunch, crunch. This shortens and strengthens the most superficial abdominal muscle, the rectus, because the muscle doesn't reach its full length on the way down. Reasons for muscles not reaching full length vary. The muscle might be tired, you could not be practicing good form, the emphasis could be on the shortened contraction, or the movements could be fast and out of control.

It's easier to work the muscles short as in a crunch. You probably can do 50 crunches, but doing 5 Roll-Ups is another story. Why? Because the focus is to work all the abdominal muscles (rectus, transversus, internal and external obliques) evenly, and in a full range of motion. If you don't lengthen and work the abdominals evenly, you get muscle imbalances—hence, muscle monster!

You won't be able to do many reps of these exercises. The emphasis is full range of motion to lengthen the muscles. Plus, you work for muscle symmetry, which is why these exercises tend to be a physical challenge even if you can bench-press a car!

Crank Up the Power!

Okay, you got it; the moves are more challenging. You need to return to the guiding principle: control. The emphasis for these 2 weeks is to engage even more muscle fibers and to crank up the brain power to make your body move the way you want it to, with control.

Here are the new moves for weeks 3 and 4: Open-Leg Rocker, Corkscrew, the Swan, Single-Leg Kick, Neck Pull, and Side-Kick Series. You're moving away from the introductory work to advance your workout. For example, after you've completed the Spine Stretch, add the Open-Leg Rocker. After that, you'll do the Corkscrew, the Saw, and so forth. You're building your Mat class workout, so practice the moves you've already learned. Here's how these exercises fit into the program to develop your body uniformly:

- The Hundred
- Roll-Up
- Hamstring Circles
- Ankle Circles
- Leg Circles
- Rolling Like a Ball
- Single-Leg Stretch
- Double-Leg Stretch
- Spine Stretch
- Open-Leg Rocker
- The Corkscrew
- The Saw
- Single-Leg Kick
- The Swan
- Child's Pose
- Neck Pull
- Side-Kick Series (see Chapter 11)
- Seal

Remember, do the exercises in order. There's a definite progression, and each move prepares you for the next, which is more challenging. Joseph Pilates brilliantly masterminded each move to work each muscle without fatigue and strain.

Open-Leg Rocker

Can you balance? Can you stay in control? The Open-Leg Rocker tests how complete you are. Finding imbalances in your body is a good thing. You may have a tendency to roll to one side if that side is stronger than the other. The goal is to roll evenly to balance the muscles of your spine and abdominals. Work them as a team to roll with balance and control.

You must scoop, scoop, scoop here. The Open-Leg Rocker is 100 percent belly! Keep your center firm, scooping harder and harder to control the roll. Remember, squeeze every ounce of air out to protect your lower back.

Go for advanced Open-Leg Rocker using these steps:

1. Sit on the mat. Scoop your pelvis to balance, and lift your legs to the ceiling to create a V, with your feet at eye level. Your legs are a little wider than your shoulders, all your limbs are straight, and your chin is on your chest.

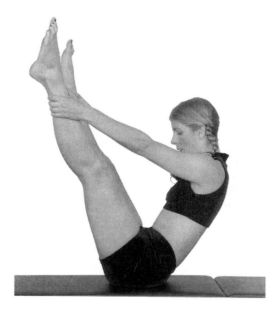

2. Inhale to roll back, making sure your weight lands on your shoulders and your head never touches the mat.

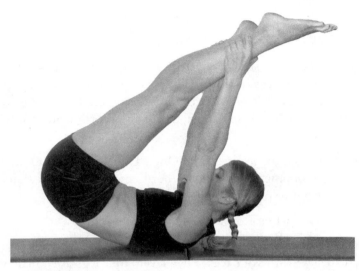

3. Exhale to roll up, and scoop to a balanced V position. If you come up too quickly or flop to one side, slightly bend your knees and tighten your tummy. It's all about focus, balance, and control. Repeat five times.

FIT FACT

In his book, *Pilates' Return to Life Through Contrology,* Joseph Pilates inhales to lift his legs up from the floor into the Open-Leg Rocker, which is very advanced. He then exhales to roll back with slow control and inhales to roll up. You can really mix up the "point of effort" and therefore switch up the breath work. For example, for more advancement—as you roll up, sit even higher up on your butt bones to really work your abs. In any event, play with it and have fun because it's a powerhouse exercise that's tons of fun no matter your level.

You can modify the Open-Leg Rocker with these steps:

1. Get in position, and wrap your arms underneath your legs to lift up your knees. Your toes should dangle just off the mat.

2. Inhale as you lift your right leg, with your toes reaching to the ceiling. Don't round your back, yet stay steady in your pelvis.

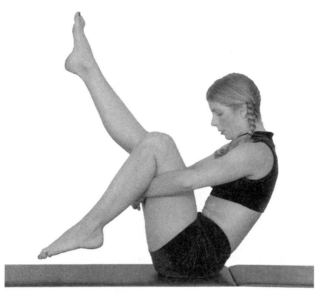

3. Exhale and lower your right leg. Inhale and lift your left leg. Again, focus on scooping to help stabilize your pelvis. Exhale and lower your left leg. Do three reps.

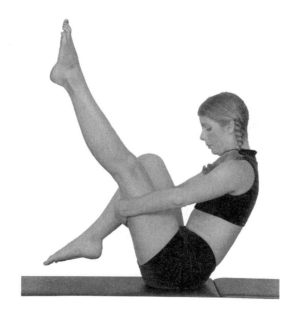

4. Inhale to straighten both legs to a V. Exhale to close the V, and inhale to reopen the V. Exhale, lowering your legs to the floor. Try this exercise four times.

FIT FACT

The Open-Leg Rocker is a great exercise that tests your coordination and strength as well as your flexibility and control in motion. You may find muscle imbalances between the left and right sides of your body. The goal is to roll evenly to balance the muscles of your spine and abdominals. Work them as a team to roll with balance and control.

The Corkscrew

The Corkscrew strengthens your deep transverse and oblique abs while challenging your trunk stability as you circle your legs as if they were one. Your limbs move from your core, so you must center before circling your legs.

There are a few different versions of the Corkscrew, but here you'll see only one.

Focus on firmness up and down your spine. The tendency is to arch your neck or back off the mat as the weight of your legs circles down. Anchor from the base of your head to your sacrum, and press the backs of your arms into the mat, palms down.

Do the Corkscrew with these steps:

1. Anchor to the mat from the back of your neck to the base of your spine. Your hands should be by your side, palms pressing into the mat for stability. Your shoulders are back and down, pits to your hips.

2. Raise your legs to the ceiling. Imagine a string pulling your toes to the ceiling, so lengthen your legs away from your hips, keeping your knees and ankles together.

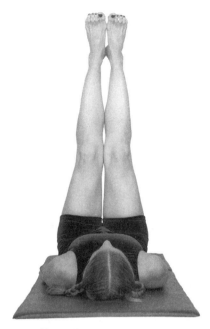

3. Inhale to make a small circle with your legs to the left, leading with your big toe and letting your right hip come off the mat slightly. Keep your knees and ankles together the entire time.

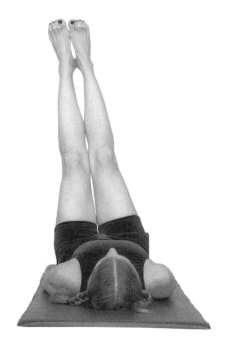

4. Exhale to complete the circle. Then reverse, and circle right and finish left. Keep the circle small to prevent you from lifting your back and neck off the mat. Repeat three to five times.

The Swan

Flip over because it's time to work your backside. Up to this point, you've worked mostly in a forward flexion, meaning abs on fire! Now, it's time to stretch your abs and work your spine. In other words, you're working your body in the opposite direction. But your abs still must work a little—in fact, you might feel a nice stretch to lengthen your look. Remember the core concepts threaded throughout all the exercises, no matter what position you're in. Therefore, even if you're on your belly, scoop your navel into your spine.

If you keep in mind the natural progression of your spine, you can redevelop your muscles, stabilize your body correctly, and perform the exercises safely. The tendency is to let your front side hang, giving no support to the delicate muscles along your spine and abdominals. Your shoulders tend to hunch toward your ears.

It's the same core concepts; you're just using them in a different direction: lift your navel to your spine, and pinch your butt cheeks to hold a $1,000 bill so you activate your pelvic floor muscles, the back of your upper thighs, and on down. Your shoulders are back and down, drawing your shoulder blades down your back. Every muscle must work, including your powerhouse.

In the prep, you'll just lift your torso and roll your head to one side and then the other. This move will help you gain strength in the muscles in your back and abs while stretching your neck muscles.

FIT FACT

Extension always starts with your head. Your body will follow.

Take flight with the Swan in these steps:

1. Lie on your stomach.

2. Place your hands directly under your shoulders, palms down. Your elbows are close to your rib cage. Stretch your toes long, as if a string is pulling on your big toe. Put some tone in your butt cheeks, lift up your navel, and press your shoulders back and down to your hips.

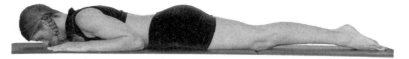

3. Inhale and slowly lift your breastbone to the ceiling, as if you're a skittish turtle not wanting to come out of your shell. Create length in the back of your neck to the base of your spine, keeping your shoulders down.

4. Keep lifting as you look at the wall—as long as you can—while pushing your palms into the mat. Think up, up, up as not to crush your vertebra. Pinch, pinch, pinch your butt cheeks. Brush your rib cage with your elbows, and keep them close to your body as your shoulder blades descend down your back.

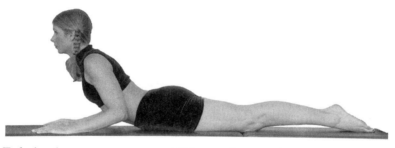

5. Exhale, drop your torso, and lift your legs at the same time, keeping your elbows by your side to control the dive. The palms of your hands support the weight of your trunk. Keep your face up, and stay lifted. It doesn't have to be a big drop; just get used to rocking on your belly button. Repeat three to five times.

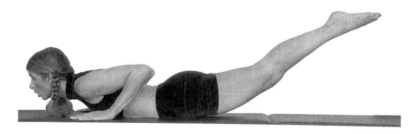

PILATES PRECAUTION

Be careful—this isn't a face drop. Don't give your dentist any more business by knocking out your two front teeth. Control your rocks by pushing and pulling with the palms of your hands, and keep your elbows glued to your rib cage.

Single-Leg Kick

Let's keep working your backside, lifting your abs and working the muscles along your spine. It's time for the Single-Leg Kick, which actually stretches your quads while you strengthen your hamstrings and gluteus.

The Single-Leg Kick is also a coordination exercise because you alternate your legs as they "kick-pulse" from left to right. The same rules apply. Put an imaginary $1,000 bill between your butt cheeks, squeeze, and press your thigh bones into the mat.

To modify this exercise, you can put a pillow underneath your belly to help support your back. If you feel any pressure in your knees, put a towel or pad underneath to cushion them.

Here's what you need to do:

1. Lie on the mat and lift your abs.

2. Squeeze your butt cheeks, and press your thigh bones into the mat. Put your elbows directly under your shoulders and toward your belly to make an upside-down V. Press your elbows into the mat.

3. Make a fist, and put your hands together. Lift your head out of your shoulders as your breastbone lifts to the ceiling so it lengthens away from your hips.

4. Inhale and draw your right heel to your butt, keeping your trunk secure and knees together.

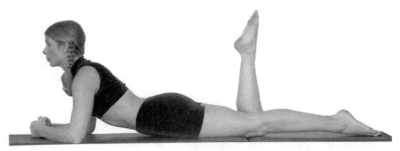

5. Pump rapidly—kick and pulse, keeping your knee pressing into the mat.

6. As you return your heel to the mat, exhale and bring your left heel up. Kick and pulse. Keep a steady rhythm going, with both legs moving at the same time. Guess what's not moving—your pelvis. No dancing hips and no butt-cheek jiggle. Do three to five sets.

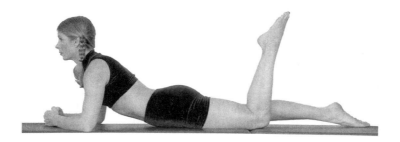

 FIT FACT

Single-Leg Kicks are snappy kicks that test your coordination. Keep kicking to establish a nice rhythm from left to right, never setting your leg down before the other leg is up—kick and pulse. Don't let your thigh bones shift from side to side—no dancing hips.

The Much-Needed Rest: Child's Pose

Your spine muscles need a rest now. Get in a position called Child's Pose, and inhale and exhale after oh-so-much work. There's nothing to it. Breathe naturally, in and out five times or so. Imagine your spine collapsing with every deep exhalation, releasing the grippers or tight muscles in your spine. Just relax and let your body wind down.

Relax in Child's Pose with these steps:

1. Slide your bottom back so it's resting on your heels. Arms go over your head or down by your side.

2. Inhale up into your spine, and exhale to pull your belly off your thighs.

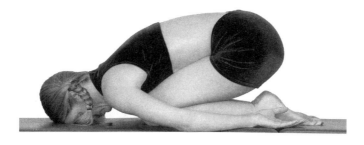

Back to the Belly: Neck Pull

Okay, back to work. Let's finish with the Neck Pull; it's another belly exercise that makes you sweat.

The good news is, you'll use the same core concepts: peeling your spine bone by bone, anchoring your spine to the mat, putting your chin to your chest, pinching your butt cheeks, and so forth. However, the Neck Pull challenges the powerhouse even more. For this exercise, imagine curling and uncurling your spine like you're opening a can of sardines.

But heed this warning: if you feel pulling in your back, start with the bent-knee modification. You'll do the same steps, only with your knees bent. Take your time with this exercise; it's definitely a gut challenge—but not at the risk to your back, please.

Fire up your abs with the Neck Pull:

1. Anchor your spine to the mat, and scoop.

2. Clasp your hands behind your head, with your elbows on the mat so you can see them from your peripheral vision. Open your legs so they're about hip-width apart. Press your heels away from your hips.

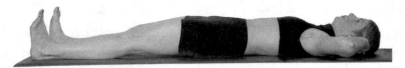

3. Inhale to lift your chin to your chest, peel your spine off the mat, and scoop. Don't hide your face as you roll up; your elbows are in your peripheral vision.

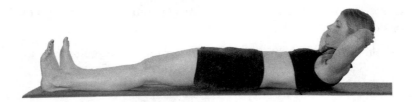

4. Exhale as you curl your nose to your belly button. Remember, glue your abs to your spine!

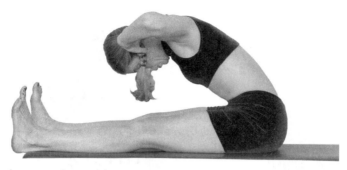

5. Inhale to stack your bones as you uncurl your head to the ceiling until you're sitting out of your hips.

6. Still inhaling, lean back into a plank position so your stomach is flat, with your heels pressing away from your hips. Pinch your butt cheeks to keep you stable.

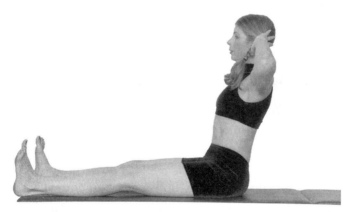

7. Exhale as you scoop to roll down bone by bone. Keep your abs as close to your back as possible, press your heels away from your hips, and squeeze your butt cheeks.

8. Press your heels away as you roll down bone by bone until the very last vertebra is between your ears. Don't plop down! Repeat three to five times.

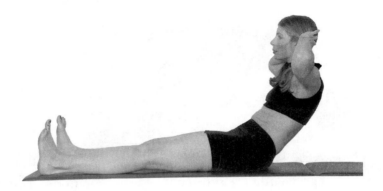

It's a Wrap

After week 4, you should definitely witness a shift. Perhaps you can almost fit into your favorite pair of jeans or your love handles are diminishing. Maybe you just feel great because you're doing something wonderful for your body. Oh yeah, squeeze, squeeze, squeeze!

The Least You Need to Know

- To change your body, you need to go slow, hold your body a little longer, and squeeze each muscle.
- You're creating a bulging monster if you do crunches only.
- Pilates exercises work your body in a full range of motion, emphasizing an eccentric contraction to create a long and strong body.
- Extension always starts with your head and then your body will follow.
- Use your breath to move your body.

Graduate to an "It" Body

In This Chapter

- Love handle–free and loving life
- Connect the moves with transitions
- Increase intensity with more challenging moves
- Seven new moves to complete the shape-up basics

If you've got it, flaunt it. But what if you lost it along the way? Can you still get it? Chiseling your curves so you can show off your body is what these last two weeks bring you. Getting the body you want may simply be a matter of taking the moves you've been doing one step further.

To get an "it" body, you gotta turn up the heat. In this chapter, you work in several new positions to recruit more muscle as you challenge your body in a few different planes of movement. You use your body in big movements to create even more resistance for your core and limbs.

Consider your body a temple; its parts work flawlessly to move in harmony so you can flaunt it.

Flaunting Your Flow

To keep your body primed, you must increase the degree of difficulty—you know this already. So in these weeks, you'll incorporate the principle of time. In fact, you'll reduce your workout time by moving through the exercises a little faster, yet never sacrificing good form. How? By focusing on the guiding principle of flow.

Think of your workout as one big dance, with movements connecting from one to another by way of a transitional move. In weeks 5 and 6, you've advanced to intermediate status. You should have exercises committed to memory: the order, the exercises, breathing patterns, and how to safely move. Running through them without stopping is icing on the cake; it's fine-tuning.

Imagine you're an Olympic competitor going for the gold. It's not enough just to know the routine. There's that something extra that distinguishes between the gold and silver medals. You're focused, executing each move with precision and control, and your routine just flows. That's your goal for these weeks: allow no wasted motion. Come prepared to perform and show off your stuff.

Here's the transition rule: if your legs finish on the floor—let's say, after Leg Circles—do a Roll-Up to the next move, which would be Rolling Like a Ball. As another example, after you complete the Fives, do a Roll-Up to get in position for the Spine Stretch.

FIT FACT

If these moves are too easy, reevaluate your form. Even in weeks 5 and 6, you should be very challenged by the exercises themselves. In addition, you're striving to embody the guiding principle: flow. You will flow from one move to another. Flow transfers into your daily life in the way of grace. Transitions between exercises are as important as the exercises themselves!

Ready, Set, Rhythm?

Have you ever tapped your foot as a song plays on the radio? That's rhythm! It's a regular succession of moves that's difficult to put into words. But it's in your body, and inevitably it will be in your Mat moves.

Certain exercises are intended to click along at a succinct pace. Just like the rap-a-tap-tap of your toes, a few moves will spur a little soul in you. Take the Side-Kick Series, for example. One leg moves gracefully into the next move, into the next, and so forth. You keep the work flowing from leg exercise to leg exercise. While rhythm is often very individual and elusive, you'll get pointers on how to move from one exercise to the next, and you'll have fun doing so.

Why rhythm? It's hard work, for one, and you're developing muscle stamina, meaning you're training your muscle to work over and over again. A body builder, for instance, will have muscle strength or the ability to lift heavy loads. Muscle stamina, though, is a more subtle strength. A boxer is a perfect example. The fact that he can throw a series of rapid-fire punches is muscle stamina. It's a way of upping the workload so your body evolves stronger and more refined. In other words, it's details. Sure, you can memorize the moves, but it's the details that make your mind and body work in harmony. No move should be just a move!

FIT FACT

Pilates trains you for life and makes you stronger for everyday movements. It improves your flexibility, coordination, muscle strength, and muscle stamina. Can you think of instances in your everyday life that require you to move in so many training modes?

If You've Got It, Flaunt It!

How will you improve your muscle endurance, develop a balanced body, and refine your body? By asking your muscles to do more. The real challenge comes from integrating several muscle groups in nontraditional ways. Instead of working just forward and back, you'll stabilize your core while lifting a leg or an arm. After all, that's how you move in real life. You squat and twist to pick up something from the floor. There are no pure exercises—all involve several muscle groups, as well as stretching and flexing to keep your body nimble and healthy.

There's always a way to increase the intensity to keep your body primed and challenged.

In these weeks, you'll add more movement, use the guiding principle of control to work your muscles instead of moving them with momentum, and you'll use flow to eliminate the rest periods between exercises. You'll also attempt to establish a nice rhythm by completing the Fives and the Side-Kick Series. In addition, you'll add new exercises: Double-Leg Kick, Shoulder Bridge (stability), Teaser 1, Swimming, and Leg Pulls.

Remember, you're striving for efficiency and control, not speed and haphazard movements. Here's the entire sequence of exercises:

- The Hundred
- Roll-Up

- Hamstring Circles
- Ankle Circles
- Leg Circles
- Rolling Like a Ball
- The Fives: Single-Leg Stretch, Double-Leg Stretch, Single Straight-Leg Stretch, Double Straight-Leg Stretch, and Crisscross
- Spine Stretch
- Open-Leg Rocker
- The Corkscrew
- The Saw
- The Swan
- Single-Leg Kick
- Double-Leg Kick
- Neck Pull
- Shoulder Bridge (stability)
- Side-Kick Series (all)
- Teaser 1
- Swimming
- Leg Pull Front
- Leg Pull Back
- Seal

ON THE MAT

Joseph Pilates invented a variety of moves to develop the whole body and all its muscles. After all, that's how we move in real life.

Love Handle–Free and Loving It: The Fives

Imagine the Energizer Bunny—it just keeps going and going and going! So will your powerhouse. It works to stabilize your trunk while you lower, lift, and scissor your legs. Just think, you can be love handle–free and loving life.

The good news is, you're almost there. After the Single- and Double-Leg Stretch, add a Single Straight-Leg Stretch, Double Straight-Leg Stretch, and Crisscross. Don't forget that if your neck muscles give out before your belly, lower your head to the mat or put one hand behind your head for support. Don't strain. To help establish a continuous tempo, focus on your breathing.

Even while pushing your powerhouse to the max, maintain butt-cheek tone. Now is a good time to introduce *push from the tush*. This push comes from a pinch in the lower tush, inner thigh, back of the thigh, and lower belly and helps to safely lift your straight legs from the floor up to the ceiling. In other words, pinching your tush provides a little extra trunk support and tones your tush.

DEFINITION

As the difficulty of the exercises increases, you'll move with utmost muscle control. Whenever you read **push from the tush,** initiate the movement from your bottom: your tush, your upper thighs, the back of your upper thighs, and your powerhouse.

The movement and breathing patterns vary from exercise to exercise, so follow the pictures.

Perform the Single Straight-Leg Stretch using these steps:

1. You're on your back, and you've just finished the Double-Leg Stretch, with your knees in to your chest.

2. Your chin on your chest lifts your shoulders off the mat. At the same time, lift one leg to the ceiling, holding your ankle or calf with both your hands while extending the other leg to the side wall, about eye level. Now pinch your butt cheeks.

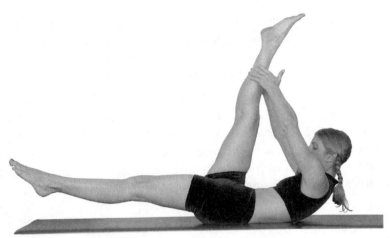

3. Inhale and pulse the lifted leg twice. Exhale and switch your legs to pulse the other leg, keeping your legs straight the whole time. Imagine scissoring your legs to establish a rapid rhythm. Don't forget to blow out every ounce of air and make your belly as flat as possible.

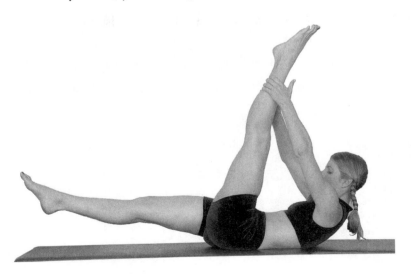

4. Repeat 5 to 10 times and then bring both your legs up to the ceiling to prepare for the Double Straight-Leg Stretch.

Perform the Double Straight-Leg Stretch using these steps:

1. As your toes lengthen out of your hip joints to the ceiling, clasp your hands behind your head for support.

2. Scoop your belly button in and up, and be heavy in your torso.

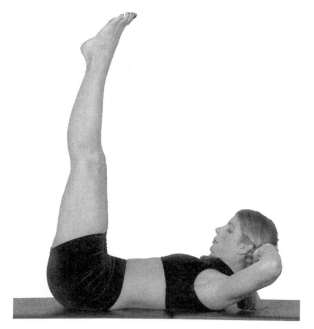

3. Inhale to lower your legs to the floor. Only take your legs as low as your back will allow. No strain, no arch, no bulge!

4. Exhale to lift your legs to the ceiling, blowing out every ounce of breath to make yourself skinny.

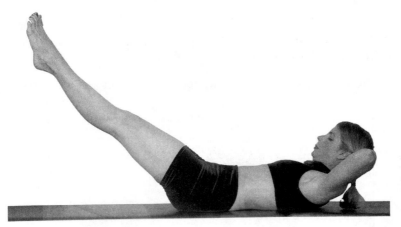

5. Push from your tush, meaning the lift initiates from your lower tush, your inner thigh, the back of your thigh, and your lower belly—scoop in and up! Do 5 to 10 raises.

6. After you're done, pull your knees in to your chest, but keep your shoulders up off the mat so you can transition into the Crisscross.

PILATES PRECAUTION

If you have lower-back problems, skip the Double Straight-Leg Stretch. Or if you'd like to try it, bend your knees to reduce some of the pressure on your lower back. In addition, keep your toes pointing toward the ceiling; the higher your legs, the less stress on your back.

Perform the Crisscross by following these steps:

1. Extend one leg about eye level, while keeping your right knee toward your chest. Lift your chin to your chest.

2. Inhale and twist your torso, with your elbow reaching to the ceiling and your armpit to your knee. Twist a little farther each time as you count to 3.

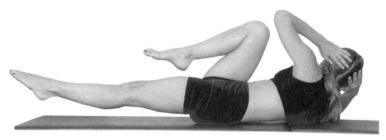

3. Exhale, and switch arms and legs. On the twist, reach as far back as you can, and keep both shoulders off the ground. Repeat 5 to 10 times.

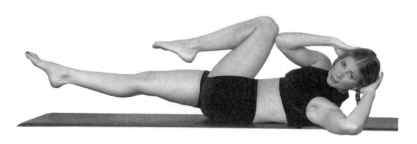

Double-Leg Kick

Got stress? Who doesn't? It will most likely affect how you hold your shoulders and upper back. The Double-Leg Kick, then, is a thorough stretch for your chest and upper back. It's also a total mental challenge because it tests your coordination skills. For example, your body moves in three different directions: your head turns as your heels draw in to your bottom, while your arms shave up and down your back.

FIT FACT

Whenever you're on your belly, don't flab it. Scoop your navel to pull your abdominals to your spine and maximize your powerhouse.

To modify this exercise, kick just your legs or do your arms only, dividing the multiple movements into one or the other. As you progress, you can put them together.

After you perform the Single-Leg Kick, do the Double-Leg Kick immediately.

Here are the steps to the Double-Leg Kick:

1. Lie on your stomach, with your right cheek on the mat—don't let your belly button touch the mat.

2. Clasp your left hand around two fingers on your right hand, and position them in the middle of your back, elbows to the floor. You should feel a nice stretch. Inhale to cue your body.

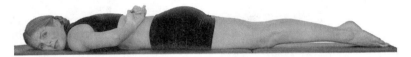

3. Exhale and draw your heels to your bottom.

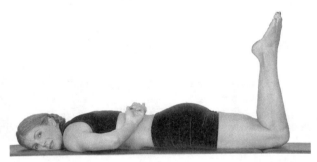

4. Pulse three times to get your hamstrings working. Be careful; don't lift your thigh bones off the mat.

5. Inhale into extension, pinching your tush while shaving your arms down your back to lift your chest off the mat. Your shoulder blades should pull together to roll your shoulders back as you lift your clasped hands toward the ceiling to ensure a good chest stretch.

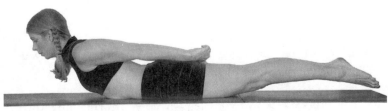

6. After that, turn your head so your other cheek touches the mat, and repeat the sequence four times.

Shoulder Bridge (Stability)

The Shoulder Bridge is a perfect example of how the mini-exercises are built into the actual move. You'll fine-tune your bottom and hamstrings along the way while stretching your quadriceps and very tight back-of-neck muscles.

For now, you'll work on stabilizing your hips and keeping your spine in neutral as you build powerhouse strength. Your trunk should remain flat and rigid while your hips stay even and stable. The tendency is for the pelvis or one hip to sink. Imagine a yardstick balancing on your thigh bones.

To build your strength, you're going to extend your leg straight out. Hold for a count of 5 and then place your leg down. But first just warm up your spine by peeling up and down.

Build your Shoulder Bridge with these steps:

1. Lie on your back, and place your feet hip-width apart as you anchor your entire foot to the mat. Anchor your elbows, your shoulders, and the back of your head. Inhale to cue your body.

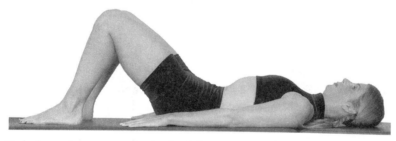

2. Exhale and scoop your abs by lifting your pubic bone to peel your spine off the mat bone by bone. Count to 5—1 Mississippi, 2 Mississippi, and so on. Inhale to imprint your spine, as if you're in the sand, to come down.

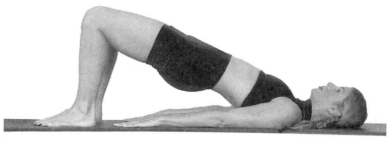

3. Repeat twice.

4. On the third time, lift one leg and hold it for a count of 5. Return the leg, and readjust your hips to lift your other leg. You're striving to keep your hips even—no sags.

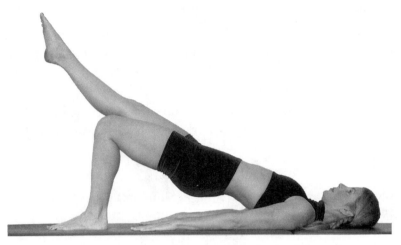

5. Repeat once. Imprint your spine, as if you're in the sand, to come down.

Teaser 1

C'mon, admit it, you're dying to test your stability and mobility while developing strength and flexibility. More than anything, though, the Teaser is a whole lot of fun. It's one of those exercises that tightens your tummy and jiggle-frees your behind. All you have to do is tighten your tummy and push from your tush in harmony as you lift your body into a perfect V.

Don't sweat it. There are many variations to prepare you.

Test your Teaser with these steps:

1. Sit on the mat, and scoop your abs to engage them to balance.

2. Wrap your arms underneath your legs to lift up your knees, with your toes dangling just off the mat. Keep your knees in the frame of your body.

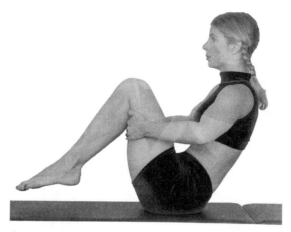

3. Inhale and raise your left leg, with your toes reaching to the ceiling. Scoop and stay steady in your pelvis.

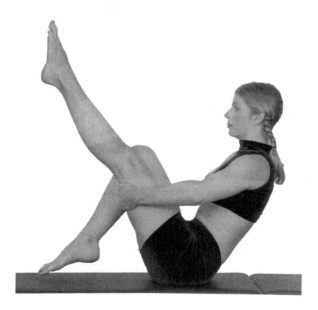

4. Exhale and lower your left leg. Repeat with the other side. Again, focus on scooping to help stabilize your pelvis.

5. Do three lifts for each leg.

6. Lift one leg up and then the other so both legs reach to the ceiling. Use your arms to support your legs, but work on your scoop to build strength and protect your back.

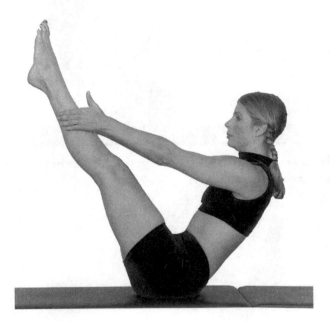

FIT FACT

The Teaser is a true test of your abdominal strength, and there are many variations of it. For example, place your feet on the wall about eye level. Inhale to lift, scooping the whole way. In addition, practice pushing from your tush. Feel the upper back of your legs and inner thighs working to bring you up. As you exhale down, push your heels against the wall to activate your hamstrings and glutes. You don't want to plop down.

Let's Go Swimming

This exercise is the perfect coordination of upper- and lower-body strength, flexibility, and balance. You must stabilize not only in your pelvis but in your shoulders as well. The tendency is for your hips to rock side to side as you lower and lift your limbs.

Think heavy in your torso, while scooping your belly button to your spine as your arms and legs move around a stable trunk. As always, draw your shoulder blades down your back to stabilize your shoulders!

As a prep, lift your right leg off the mat and also your left arm. Lift from your quadriceps to work your lower-back muscles while reaching your fingertips out in front of you. Think yourself long as you fire the hamstrings, glutes, and lower-back muscles. Don't hunch your shoulders; stabilize by drawing your shoulder blades down your back. Hold for five counts, and then reverse limbs. After you feel comfortable with lowering and lifting your limbs, go for a swim.

Go Swimming with these steps:

1. Lie on your belly.

2. Lift your limbs off the mat.

3. Follow this rhythm: inhale for five beats as you quickly alternate your arms and legs, lifting your torso a little.

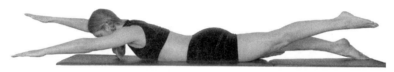

4. Then exhale for five beats as you alternate your arms and legs, lowering your torso. Your pelvis is stable, and your head will come up, with the extension of your spine following the line of your spine at all times.

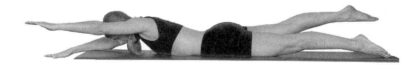

Head to Heel Like Steel: Leg Pulls

Here's your mantra: head to heel like steel. Say it over and over again. These exercises challenge your total body strength: upper and lower body, plus core stability. Not only will you stabilize your pelvis and shoulders, squeeze your butt cheeks, and press your navel to your spine, but you also have to do this in midair. At this stage, you're scooping your abs to your spine and keeping 'em in place to develop enough strength to hold yourself up. Your head and toes will be in one straight line.

However, there are rewards: firm butt, flat belly, sleek arms, while also stretching all the right places.

Here's a warning, though: depending on your strength or weakness, one hip may sink. Try to keep your hips even to establish pelvic stability. Likewise, your belly must not sag in the Leg Pull Front. When you flip over to do the Leg Pull Back, on the other hand, you must not droop your fanny. You must stay head to heel like steel, in a straight line, to benefit from these exercises.

FIT FACT

Think head, neck, spine, hips, and legs in line the whole time when performing the Leg Pulls. Keep your body in a straight line as your navel presses to your spine—no belly bulge.

For a modified Leg Pull Front, get into the same position but distribute your body weight on your elbow and toes. You can modify the Leg Pull Back the same way, balancing your body weight on your elbows and heels.

Strengthen the Leg Pull Front with these steps:

1. Lie face down on the mat.

2. Press yourself up so you're in a push-up position, with your arms directly under your shoulders.

3. Work to stabilize your hips, pull your navel to your spine, and pull your pits to your hips as you hold your body in a straight line. Also press your heels toward the back wall, and keep your head to the front wall to work in opposition to keep the middle taut. Don't sag in your belly; imagine a sharp needle is in line with your belly button. If you sag, ouch! Stay lean and in a tight, straight line. Repeat three to five times.

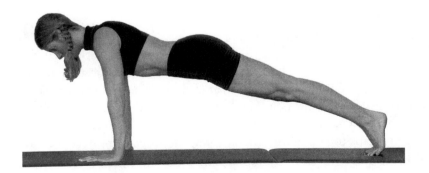

PILATES PRECAUTION

If you have any wrist or shoulder problems, be careful with the Leg Pull Front and Leg Pull Back. If you have a wrist problem, you may want to work in a neutral wrist position, for example. If you have any pain, don't do the Leg Pulls.

Develop the Leg Pull Back with these steps:

1. Flip over.

2. Place your arms shoulder width apart, with your fingertips either facing your heels or out to the side a little. Use the back of your legs to lift your bottom off the mat, keeping your body weight traveling toward your heels.

3. Squeeze your butt cheeks, and reach your legs out of your hips to make a straight line from shoulders to toes. Don't let your tush sink. Think of a string pulling you up from your belly button, yet don't bulge your belly. Keep firm in your center.

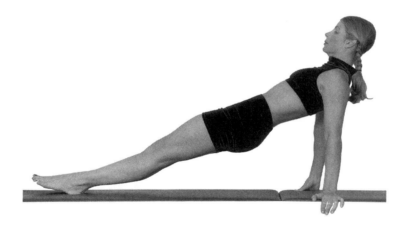

The Finish Line

Congratulations! You've just completed the 6-week Mat workout, which covers basic and intermediate moves. These exercises will challenge you for some time, so stay here and work on the moves to perfect your form. Focus on precision one week, control another, and so forth.

Remember, it's the details that make the move. Without details, moves are just moves. Why move through life when you can flaunt it?

The Least You Need to Know

- Pilates is all about movement. Don't forget to flow from exercise to exercise in your Mat workout. Add the Roll-Up as a transition into the next move so the sequence of exercises keeps flowing.
- To increase the intensity of your workout, reduce the time, increase the difficulty of the moves, and challenge your muscles not to stop.
- Pilates trains your muscles so they're prepared to live out everyday activities.
- Week 6 completes the shape-up basics, or beginner and intermediate work.

Moving On Up

Part 3 challenges you and provides enough workouts for a lifetime. In the first two chapters, you learn the advanced Mat exercises. As you get more efficient with the introductory work, you can turn to these chapters to challenge your body with moves that call for more strength, coordination, balance, flexibility, and control.

You also learn the entire Side-Kick Series, which will transform your legs and de-droop and de-dimple your bottom line. Finally, you can de-jiggle your arm waddle with exercises from the Standing Arms Series.

Smart Sweating

In This Chapter

- Buff your dimples
- Putting an edge on the shape-up basics
- Theory of opposition
- Principle of self-resistance

Attention challenge-seekers: you're headed into the final stretch. Are you feeling stronger and more energetic, even—dare I say it—breaking a sweat? No, not a pink-faced, dripping sweat. Just a little dewy under the arms and around your forehead.

A good sweat has many values. Besides detoxifying the body, it's a sign you're working hard enough to condition your muscles, including your heart. A good sweat means your intensity level is challenging enough to buff your body—even your dimples.

There's a great slogan: buff your dimples! So give up the antisweat dreams. In the end, a great body is really a matter of simple math—burn more calories than you take in. A little sweat is a sign that the caloric burn is heating up.

In this chapter, you'll add more intensity to some of the exercises you've already done plus learn a few new super-advanced moves, making your workout a bit harder. Yet you'll get the body you want and bask in a sense of accomplishment as you almost reach the sweaty Mat finish line.

Boosting Your Ability

Reach your head out of your neck as you lengthen your toes away from your waist. It's subtle nuances like these that turn up your internal furnace a few degrees to burn more calories. Think *theory of opposition*, which is a way to move your body in two different directions.

DEFINITION

The **theory of opposition** moves the body in two different directions to engage more muscle groups. It increases the resistance of all the exercises and gets you in touch with your body.

As the Mat exercises increase in difficulty, you must develop a certain awareness of how your body moves and muscles work. In other words, you're boosting your ability to fine-tune.

A Roll-Up works deep abdominal muscles—and that's probably where you felt most of the work up to this point. When you work with opposition, not only will you use the muscles of your belly, but you also will use your hamstrings and inner thighs. You're learning to better control your movement and activate as many muscle groups as possible.

As the moves increase in intensity, you must work in opposition. Let's take a closer look at the Roll-Up:

Opposition 1: As you peel off the mat, bone by bone, you'll press your heels away from your hips to activate your hamstrings. Your bottom is heavy, pulling down as your torso lifts upward. Stop here. Pushing your heels away from your hips counterbalances the weight of your trunk as it peels off the mat. Your deep abs are contracting, and so are your hamstrings as your body moves in a stable way. Hence, your body is moving in two different directions to control the move.

Opposition 2: As you complete the Roll-Up, reach your fingertips long past your toes while your belly button pulls your abdominals back toward your spine. Translation: as your fingertips reach forward, so do your heels. Your belly pulls back so your body moves in two different directions—your deep abs contract as your hamstrings stretch.

Opposition 3: As your fingers reach past your toes, your pelvis moves into a scoop to continue to challenge your deep abs. Then you'll press your heels away from your hips to roll down bone by bone to engage your hamstrings; pinch your butt cheeks. This weight in your bottom and heels gets your hamstrings contracting so you have better control of the roll, and this prevents you from plopping down.

Control is crucial; it's safer, therefore, to work in opposition. If you roll down without pressing your heels away from your hips, your hamstrings and inner thighs don't get a workout—and, worse, your legs may lift off the mat, shattering your anchored position. You could get injured.

Tackling the Next Level

You've probably been doing just fine yet felt a little overwhelmed. After all, there are many exercises, breathing techniques, core concepts, and guiding principles to think about. By far, theory of opposition is one of the more difficult concepts to grasp. Nevertheless, incorporate it so you get the most out of your workout: control, concentration, flow, and precision of movement.

Body awareness helps you move with control and precision. This resistance, in return, turns up the caloric burn. Being in touch with your body and how it moves while exercising is the best gift you can give yourself.

FIT FACT

Everything works in opposition: man, woman, sun, moon, winter, and summer. Our muscles, too, come in pairs that work in opposition; it's the key to life. When we work in opposition—with two ends working away from each other—we keep the middle taut. If your legs relax, your middle sags; if your arms release energy, your middle sags, too.

Before tackling the new moves, try the Mat exercises you already know in opposition. I guarantee you'll work that much harder. You'll find you have more control and better form, and you'll ultimately engage more muscles. As you put this theory to the test, pay attention to the muscle groups that come into play. Of course, you'll reap all the usual benefits, but this extra challenge definitely tightens your look. Precision, focus, and control never meant sweat free.

What's Next?

Remeasure! Rejump to check your jiggles! Don't step on the scale, though. Instead, your goal is to cut an inch, have fewer jiggles, or have extra room in your trousers. So take out the tape measure and evaluate your makeover progress. Be realistic, though. Don't expect a mega-reduction in inches; however, an inch is an impressive start.

Take this time to set new goals and write them down. You may want to take another set of pictures. You're shooting for another 6 weeks before remeasuring again.

There's no rush to add these exercises. They're super-advanced and are often done in an Advanced Mat class. You can continue to do the Mat work you've already learned for months. Working in opposition will put a new spin on the movements.

When you're ready, however, the new exercises are as follows: the Rollover, Spine Twist, the Jackknife, and Push-Ups. Then there are the advanced versions of some moves you learned earlier: The Swan, Shoulder Bridge, Leg Pull Front and Back, and the Teaser. You're definitely not missing a muscle.

Here's the entire sequence of exercises:

- The Hundred
- Roll-Up
- Rollover
- Hamstring Circles
- Ankle Circles
- Leg Circles
- Rolling Like a Ball
- The Fives: Single-Leg Stretch, Double-Leg Stretch, Single Straight-Leg Stretch, Double Straight-Leg Stretch, and Crisscross
- Spine Stretch
- Open-Leg Rocker
- The Corkscrew
- The Saw
- The Swan

- Single-Leg Kick
- Double-Leg Kick
- Neck Pull
- Shoulder Bridge (kicks)
- Spine Twist
- The Jackknife
- Side-Kick Series (see Chapter 11)
- Teaser
- Swimming
- Leg Pull Front (kicks)
- Leg Pull Back (kicks)
- Seal
- Push-Ups

Control Is Crucial: The Rollover

This exercise tests your spine's flexibility. It also works your deep abs and back muscles as you roll down bone by bone. You might even feel a little stretch in your hamstrings as you articulate the length of your spine. The Rollover tests your opposition. Picture this: as your legs go over your head, glue your abs to your spine the whole time—legs one way, abs the other.

The Rollover requires a tremendous amount of belly strength, so don't be surprised if you can't lift your hips over your head. Try this modification: follow the same directions but make a diamond with your legs. Inhale to lift your hips over your head; exhale to roll down bone by bone. Repeat three to five times. Do this prep until you get enough strength to lift your legs over your head, as shown in the pictures.

The movement is a little tricky. You'll start with the legs closed. Roll over and then open the legs to roll down. Reverse the leg sequence; open and close to roll down the spine as if a string of pearls is hitting the mat one at a time.

PILATES PRECAUTION

If you have had any neck or upper-back problems, skip this exercise. In addition, if you have high blood pressure or a condition called macular degeneration, you should not do any moves that put too much pressure on your head, the Rollover and the Jackknife, specifically.

Perform your Rollover with these steps:

1. Lie on your back with your hands by your side, palms down.

2. You have two options for your legs: lengthen your toes to the ceiling to anchor your tailbone to the mat, which is slightly easy; or, for a super challenge, start with straight legs on the mat. However, you must have enough belly strength to keep your back anchored to the mat at all times.

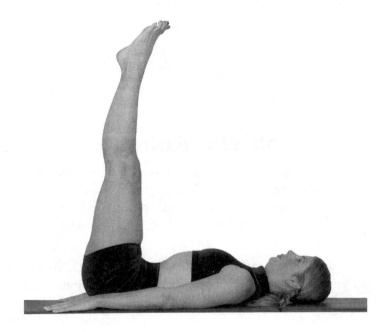

3. In one movement, inhale to engage your abs and push from your tush to lift your hips over your head, keeping your legs closed. Hover your toes a few inches off the mat, keeping your knees directly over your eyes. Reach your fingertips long so the weight of your body doesn't land on your neck. Notice the scoop!

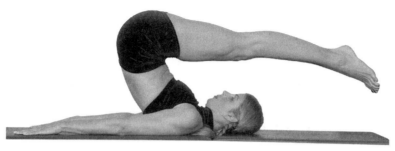

4. Exhale to open your legs just past your shoulders.

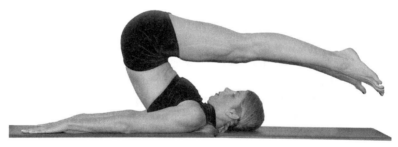

5. Inhale to roll down your spine bone by bone, and feel each bone as it lengthens your spine. Control the roll four ways: press the back of your arms into the mat, lengthen your toes away from your hips so the weight of your bottom doesn't pull you down, reach your fingertips long as you roll down, and keep scooping.

6. Exhale as you bring your legs to the floor.

7. When your tailbone touches the mat, either stop or continue to lower your legs to the mat. Stop only if you can keep your back flat on the mat—*only!* If you can't, just lower your legs until your back can safely remain flat on the mat and then push from your tush and squeeze your upper thighs to lift your legs back over your head again.

8. Do three sets with your legs closed and then another three with your legs open, for a total of six.

FIT FACT

All these exercises move in opposition to add more resistance so your body works a little harder, to work your body with control, and to protect your body from injury. Moving in opposition takes the exercises to the next level—precision, control, focus!

Hush Your Hips: Shoulder Bridge (Kicks)

Now you're ready to add some kicks to the Shoulder Bridge, which, of course, cranks up the intensity. The goal is to kick and keep your trunk completely still. As Joseph Pilates said, "Quiet hips." When you kick your leg to the ceiling, the tendency is for your hips to sink. Instead, imagine that a sling hangs from the ceiling to hoist your hips to prevent your bottom from sinking into the mat. Resist by pressing the foot of your standing leg into the mat as if you're pushing your hips up as well. To refresh your memory, the Shoulder Bridge works all the right areas: your powerhouse, glutes, hamstrings, and inner thighs.

Kick start your Shoulder Bridge with these steps:

1. Lie on your back. Set your feet hip-width apart as you anchor your entire foot to the mat. Anchor your elbows, shoulders, and the back of your head. Scoop your pubic bone to lift your spine off the mat bone by bone. Stretch out a leg in front of you.

2. Inhale to kick it to the ceiling.

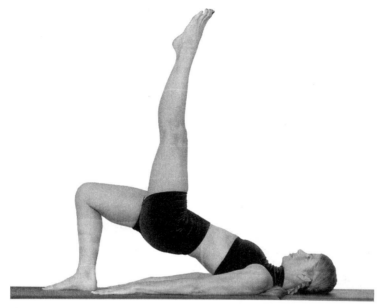

3. Exhale as the leg comes down, reaching the toes away from your hips. You can flex your foot for added bonus. Don't droop your bottom, and stay firm in your trunk. Do three to five kicks with one leg and then switch legs.

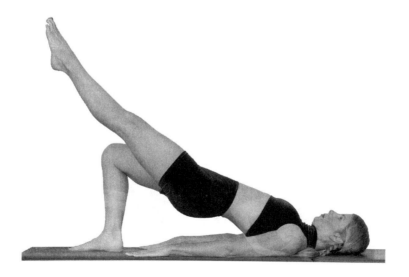

It's a Stretch: Spine Twist

Here's a treat! The Spine Twist is a breathing exercise to detoxify the bad air out of your body, plus it's a spine-soother. However, it's not as easy as it looks. As you rotate your spine, concentrate on cementing your body from your hips down. The tendency is for you to shift your hips as you twist, so focus on remaining stable.

> **ON THE MAT**
>
> Your lungs are like a sponge. Squeeze out the dirty water to let the clean water in. In the Spine Twist, squeeze out the dirty air and let the good air come in.

The "twist" is similar to the Saw. Lift up out of your hips, turn your belly button, and twist. Remember to pinch, lift, and grow! Stay anchored from the base of your spine to the very top of your head. Finally, grow your fingertips long from your arms as you twist each time. That's how you'll get the delicious spine stretch.

Soothe your spine with the Spine Twist using these steps:

1. Sit on the mat, and pinch, lift, and grow! Extend your legs long in front, with your heels and hips glued together and your feet flexed.

2. Think heavy in your tush, as if you're anchored in cement from your hips down. Extend your arms out to your sides as you reach your fingertips long. Inhale to lift up out of your hips.

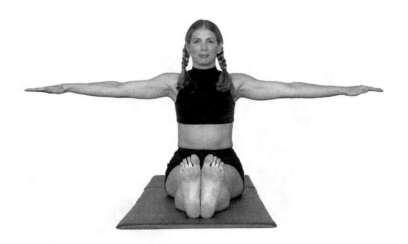

3. Turn your head to see your wrist, exhale, and twist, pulsing two times to ring the dirty air out of your lungs. Inhale to return to the center to exhale and twist the other way. Do three to five sets.

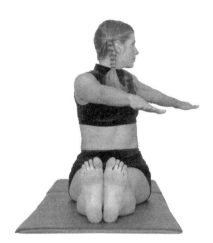

Straight as a Pencil: The Jackknife

Power up your powerhouse! The Jackknife is the ultimate test of powerhouse strength as you stretch the muscles in your neck, back, and shoulders. The Jackknife is similar to the Rollover; it challenges you to work bone by bone, only from a shoulder stand position.

The movement must be done with the utmost concentration, control, and flow. Imagine a constant flow with your legs—over your head, to the ceiling, and down to the floor. Be careful, and don't jerk yourself up or let yourself plop down. Use your powerhouse to guide you down. The challenge is to keep your feet directly over your eyes as you roll down—now that's powerhouse strength!

Generate the Jackknife with these steps:

1. Lie flat on the mat, with your legs extended out in front of you.

2. Press the back of your arms into the mat, palms down.

3. In one flowing motion, inhale to lift your legs over your head, pushing from your tush and squeezing your butt cheeks and upper inner thighs. Think Saran Wrap!

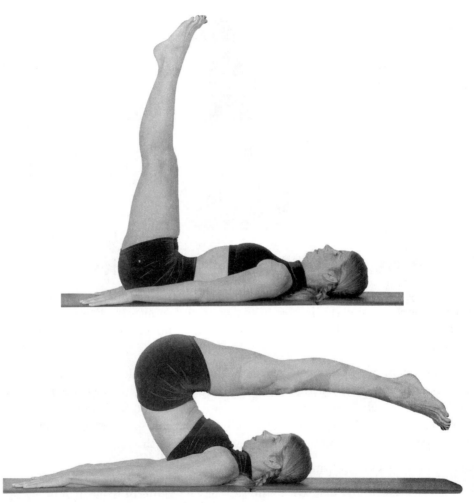

4. Lift your hips up to the ceiling, pinching your butt cheeks, to a shoulder stand. Keep pinching so you have that little extra lift. Pinch your butt, and your pelvis pushes forward to lift you into almost a straight line from your shoulders to your toes.

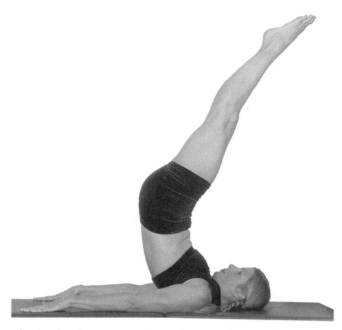

5. Press the back of your arms into the mat for support. Be careful, and stop if you feel any pressure in your neck. Exhale as you roll down, keeping your toes directly over your eyes as you roll bone by bone. Keep them reaching to the ceiling as if someone is holding your big toes!

6. Reach your fingers away from your shoulders for support, and use your powerhouse.

7. Finish by lengthening your legs to the floor. Repeat three to six times.

Not Just Any Only Old Teaser: Advanced Teaser

Up to now, you've been practicing. Good, because you need powerhouse strength for the Advanced Teaser. If not, go back to the basics so you avoid hurting your back. For example, you might pop yourself up, inadvertently straightening your back in the process, which may cause injury. Instead, push from your tush to help you up. Pinch your butt cheeks, squeeze the backs of your upper thighs, and scoop your abs, keeping 'em contracted on the way up and on the way down.

Test your Advanced Teaser with these steps:

1. Lie flat on the mat, with your legs extended out in front of you. Lengthen your arms to the ceiling (as shown) or straighten your arms overhead if you can maintain a flat back.

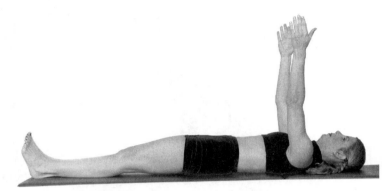

2. Inhale to bring your arms and legs up simultaneously to make a V—fold yourself like a taco! Reach your fingertips to your toes and then to your ears, keeping your abs engaged so your torso never moves.

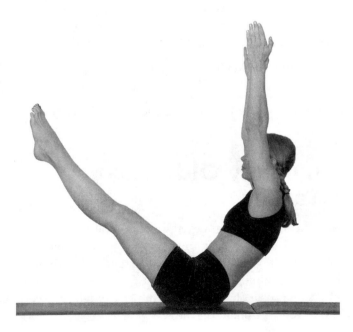

3. Exhale to unfold the V, scooping the whole way down to the mat. Repeat three to five times.

Head to Heel Like Steel: Leg Pulls (Kicks) and Push-Ups

Head to heel like steel, again! This time, you have kicks involved. After the stabilization work, you should have enough powerhouse strength to add a little extra oomph! Plus, you'll feel a nice stretch in the back of your calves.

Remember, you don't want to move your hips—keep them even and suspended.

Create the Leg Pull Front with these steps:

1. Lie face down on the mat.

2. Press yourself up into a push-up position. Glue your abs to your spine—no belly flab! The palms of your hands are directly under your shoulders.

3. Press your shoulders down, pits to your hips. Stay lean and tight in a straight line.

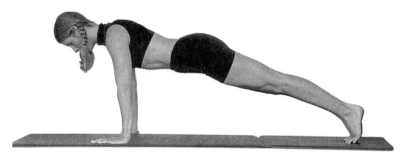

4. Inhale to lift your leg to the ceiling while simultaneously rocking your other heel back and forth; it's a rhythmic motion on the ball of the foot.

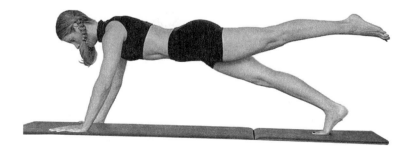

5. Exhale to put your leg down. Keep your head in line with your spine the whole time. Don't sag your belly; imagine a needle in line with your belly button—ouch! Repeat three sets of kicks.

PILATES PRECAUTION

If you have a wrist injury or a shoulder problem, skip these exercises. Or try to work with your wrist in a neutral position, perhaps making a fist and performing these on your elbows. In any event, use caution with these exercises.

Going the Other Way: Leg Pull Back (Kicks)

Now stabilize your hips going the opposite way—again the ultimate core strengthener! This time, you'll kick your leg to the ceiling. As you kick up, stay firm in your center to stabilize your body. As your leg comes down, resist gravity and the weight of your leg by pushing your hips up. To get an additional stretch in the back of your leg, lead with your heel as you lower your foot.

Strengthen the Leg Pull Back with these steps:

1. Sit on your bottom.

2. Place your arms a little wider than your shoulders, fingertips facing your butt or out to the side a little.

3. Lift your behind off the mat. Squeeze your butt cheeks and lengthen your legs out of you to make a straight line from your shoulders to your toes. Press your heels into the mat without any movement from your torso.

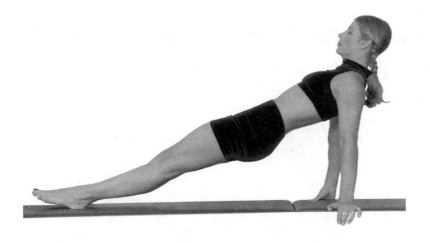

4. Inhale and kick your leg up to the ceiling.

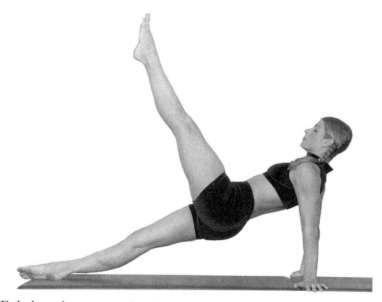

5. Exhale to lower your leg. Inhale and kick again.

6. Repeat the kick three times and then switch legs.

FIT FACT

You can add flexing and pointing your foot for an extra challenge.

A Different Class of Push-Up

Everyone hates push-ups, but you won't hate this Push-Up! It's fun, and it tightens and tones just about every muscle. Of course, this Push-Up is a little different; it's a triceps Push-Up. You won't be missing a muscle: chest, shoulders, back, triceps, legs, and powerhouse while stretching. Engage your powerhouse fully; imagine a needle shooting through your belly button if it sags.

> **FIT FACT**
>
> The Push-Up is a perfect example of Joseph Pilates' brilliance. He took the traditional push-up, which primarily uses the chest muscles, and developed a Push-Up that calls for just about every muscle in the body while your legs still get a good stretch.

If you can't get into proper Push-Up position, you have two options: do Push-Ups on the wall or on your hands and knees.

1. Stand up, feet in the Pilates V.

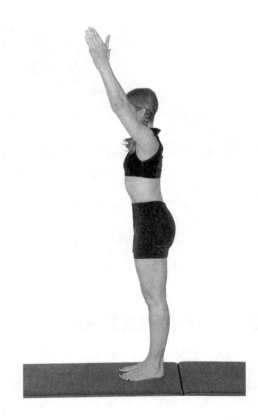

2. Inhale and walk your hands down your legs in three counts, scooping the entire time.

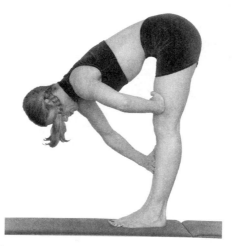

3. Exhale to walk your hands out in three counts—still scooping—so your palms are directly under your shoulders.

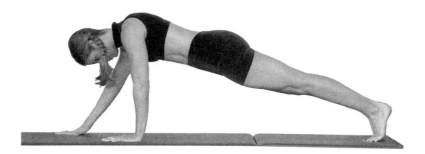

4. Remember, head to heel like steel as the crown of your head reaches long while your heels reach long in the other direction. (Use a neutral fists position if you have a wrist problem.)

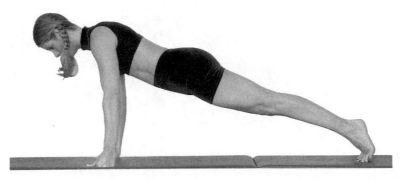

5. Inhale, bend your elbows, and lower your chest to the ground, shaving your elbows along your ribs. Keep your elbows close to your sides. Don't lift your shoulders to your ears.

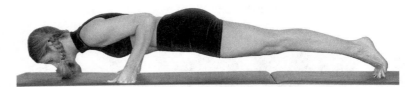

6. Exhale to push up. Imagine squeezing a pencil underneath your armpits as you push up to help stabilize your shoulders. Do three Push-Ups and then walk your hands in.

7. Roll up, scooping your abs to protect your lower back, to a standing position. Repeat three times.

FIT FACT

For the super-advanced Push-Up, you can initiate the movement with one leg. It's the same steps, but you're balancing on only one leg as you go through the sequence. The tricky part is when you come up. You must use your powerhouse to balance your leg as you lift your torso up from the floor in one shift motion. Imagine a pendulum.

Now look in the mirror and say, "I've done a *wonderful* thing for my body." That's how you'll end your Mat workout.

Be the Boss of Your Body

The goal: turn up the burn. Taking the Mat to the next level does this. You don't, however, have to add any more moves until you're good and ready. Remember, a move is just a move; anyone can memorize movements. The real work begins when you feel the exercise in your body and see it in your mind.

Be proud of your progress because you're teaching your body to obey your mind. Keep going—you're almost to the Mat finish line. And remember, scoop, length, squeeze, and pinch!

The Least You Need to Know

- A good sweat detoxifies your body and shows that you're working your muscles.
- Think theory of opposition—it's moving your body in two different ways.
- All the exercises work in opposition to increase the intensity, keep the movement safe, and control the movement.
- Joseph Pilates was a big fan of self-resistance.

The Intelligent Workout

In This Chapter

- Use your breath to quiet your mind
- Integrate your mind and body
- Visualize first
- Super-advanced moves

You can't bend and twist your body into these moves without getting your brain involved. The Mat requires patience and uninterrupted concentration. It will challenge your physical limits, but it will bolster your will as well. The workout can be spiritual, holistic, and much more. Get in touch with that mind and body awareness that continues to propel you to the next level, and the next time, and then for a lifetime.

Body and Mind Integration

Distractions can destroy concentration. Yet it's your mind that creates most of the noise—the internal noise, at least. However, you can learn how to turn off your thoughts and control your emotions with a mental training strategy called imagery. Elite athletes use imagery and visualization techniques to help them get ready for competition. So will you—not for competition, but to help you focus. After all, that's what focus is; it's clearing the mind so no thoughts, emotions, or distractions take away from your ability to perform.

Think about how you see images. Close your eyes. Imagine you're doing a Roll-Up. Can you mentally describe the steps and how your body feels while going through the move? This will help you get your mind involved so you take your workout to a higher level. You need to focus on whether you see, hear, or feel the movement; it's best if you can get as many senses involved as possible.

Do you experience the exercises from within, seeing yourself performing them? Or do you see it through images? Both are equally important. Eventually you'll need to feel the exercises from within, even if you're not doing the moves. For now, you can rely on the mental images of the photos in the exercises to get you to that point. Try the following exercise to help your imagery.

Sit in a quiet room or space. Close your eyes, and visualize the Roll-Up. Move slowly, smoothly, and with full awareness and concentration moment to moment. If your mind wanders from the move—say, you're wondering what's for dinner—bring it back. Talk to yourself. Use verbal phrases and mental imagery to regain your focus. Repeat slowly in a monotone voice the core concepts. In your head, say "scoop" or "length" or "pinch." Focus on the word you choose, and repeat it every time your mind wanders.

Give your mind vivid details: scoop by gluing your abs to your spine. Feel this sensation by pulling your belly button in and up to your spine so it's under your rib cage. The object is to use as many senses as possible so the mental picture is vivid and complete. With that, the mind can better tell the body what to do.

For the next practice run, sit in a quiet room and watch yourself performing the Roll-Up, using your breaths this time. Notice how your muscles feel when you're breathing. If your mind wanders, bring it back with your breath. Smooth, rhythmic, harmonious breathing, along with mental tuning, helps you develop a much higher level of concentration. It could be because the center for breathing is located in a part of the brain where your body's lifelines are located: the controls for muscle tone, heart movement, blood circulation, and concentration. As we know, the breath can affect heart rate, blood pressure, and the nervous system. With fast, erratic breaths, your mind becomes scattered, while deep, rhythmic breaths can calm your mind.

FIT FACT

Elite athletes must control negative thoughts, pregame jitters, and the emotional highs and lows of competition to perform well; it's done with imagery and breath control. You're no different. No, you won't be trying out for the Olympics, but you've got business deals and projects to conquer.

You've probably noticed that when you intensely focus on something, you hold your breath. For example, as the intensity level of the Mat exercises increases, your mind might get fixed on one point, perhaps causing it to wander, making you think, *I can't do this move* or *I look so stupid.* You're probably holding your breath as these negative thoughts float in and out. To erase negative thoughts, return to your breaths to keep you moving when you get stuck in negativity.

Practice makes perfect. Joseph Pilates designed each exercise with breaths so you can work toward integrating your mind and body. Before each move, use imagery to cue your mind, and use the breaths to prepare your body. Do the exercise first in your head and then move the body.

That doesn't preclude you from extra practice. You can practice imagery just before going to bed to refine your Mat technique, for example. Yet imagery and breath control are also useful strategies for everyday life. You can mentally prepare yourself to tackle a new work project or use breath control for those very stressful days. We can all benefit from learning how to control the emotional highs and lows of life.

See It and Then Do It!

Congratulations! You've entered super-advanced territory. Get ready to challenge your body to the max while engaging your mind for help. Switch the focus from the actual move to moving in your mind. Use imagery and your breath to cue your mind and keep it focused if it wanders. Pay attention to how your body feels while setting up the move and also how it feels while executing it.

FIT FACT

Use your breath to move from within. By utilizing slow, rhythmic, and harmonious breathing, you can obtain a higher level of concentration and focus.

You can add these exercises when you feel ready. You don't have to tackle them all at once. For example, you might start by adding just the Scissors and the Bicycle to your existing program. Still, you don't have to add these exercises at all, ever. You can stick to the basics for years to come and keep your body in great shape. There's always a way to challenge yourself a little more, something new to learn or a new way to feel it in your body and your mind.

Here are the last eight moves: Swan Dive, the Scissors, the Bicycle, Hip Circles, Kneeling Side Kicks, the Mermaid, the Twist, and the Boomerang.

Follow the sequence of exercises in order:

- The Hundred
- Roll-Up
- Rollover
- Hamstring Circles
- Ankle Circles
- Leg Circles
- Rolling Like a Ball
- The Fives
- Spine Stretch
- Open-Leg Rocker
- The Corkscrew
- The Saw
- The Swan Dive
- Single-Leg Kick
- Double-Leg Kick
- Neck Pull
- The Scissors
- The Bicycle
- Shoulder Bridge
- Spine Twist
- The Jackknife
- Side-Kick Series (see Chapter 11)
- Teaser
- Can-Can
- Hip Circles
- Swimming

- Leg Pull Front
- Leg Pull Back
- Kneeling Side Kicks
- The Mermaid
- The Twist
- The Boomerang
- Seal
- Push-Ups

The Swan Dive

Let's start with a Swan. Do two to three Swan preps to warm up your back muscles and then try the Swan Dive. The directions are the same, but your arms don't touch the floor. The goal is to stay rigid in your body, keep your legs glued together, and lengthen your arms to the ceiling as you rock on your belly.

Visualize and feel your abs glued to your spine, which is especially important. Scooping protects the muscles along your spine; it doesn't take much to strain them—especially if you're rocking out of control. Pinching your butt cheeks also helps control the rock. Remember: muscle, not momentum!

 PILATES PRECAUTION

Attention, men: the Swan Dive may cause a little discomfort to your privates as you rock. You may need to put a pad or pillow under your hips—perhaps near your thigh bones or whatever is comfortable for you.

Rock the Swan Dive with these steps:

1. Lie on your stomach.

2. Place your hands directly under your shoulders, palms down, with your elbows glued to your rib cage.

3. Reach your toes long, as if a string is pulling your big toes.

4. Pinch your butt cheeks, scoop your navel to your spine, and press your shoulders back and down.

5. Inhale to straighten your arms and lift your head, neck, shoulders, and breast-bone off the floor.

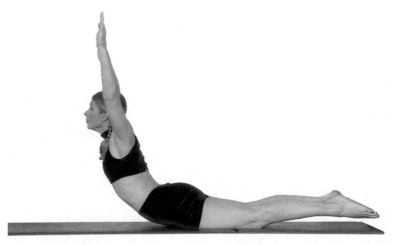

6. Exhale to lift your hands and drop your torso. As you rock, extend your arms out in front of you.

7. As you rock up, tighten your back as if your shoulder blades are drawing down your back, and lift from your back. Pinch as your legs go up, and scoop. Feel length in your body as you reach. Repeat five times.

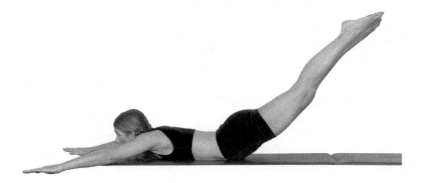

ON THE MAT

In *Pilates' Return to Life Through Contrology,* Joseph writes to stay rigid and lift your legs off the mat as you lift your chest high off the mat.

Age-Defying Moves: The Scissors and the Bicycle

Maintain quiet hips in these two exercises. Core stability is so important; nothing moves but your legs.

Here's your first set of age-defying moves. The sequence starts with the Scissors and the Bicycle. The moves are rhythmic and nonstop, so you must correctly set up the movement before using your legs. Scoop your abs and turn on your powerhouse to stabilize your trunk. Think about the opposition: lengthen your leg to the front as your other leg lengthens behind you—imagine you're doing a split on the ceiling.

Press your shoulders, elbows, and the base of your skull into the floor for a solid base of support. As your legs move, your body presses up, defying gravity, as your legs go in opposition. Very little or no weight is placed on your wrists and elbows.

You've got to scoop and pinch your heart out to keep your body still as your legs move; it's a trial of core stability, strength, and coordination. Plus, your bottom is getting a workout.

The Scissors

Split your Scissors with these steps:

1. Lie flat on your back, and lift your tush over your head, squeezing the backs of your upper thighs. Lead with your pelvis—keep pinching your butt cheeks so your toes reach long to the ceiling. At the same time, place the palms of your hands on your lower back so your bottom rests in your hands.

2. Anchor the back of your arm, from the elbow to your shoulder, to the mat. Stay firm, scoop, and pinch your butt cheeks; it's this connection between your abs and glutes that stabilizes you as well.

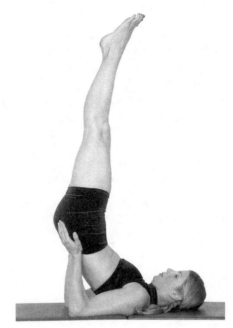

3. In a split movement, inhale to lengthen one leg to the front while the other leg reaches past your head.

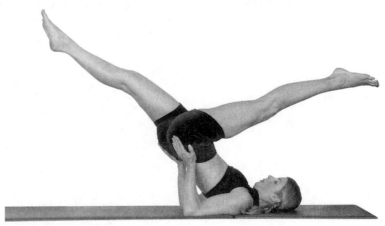

4. Exhale to switch legs in a scissorslike motion. After three sets of scissors, go right into the Bicycle.

ON THE MAT

Joseph says: "Keep body rigid, move legs only .... Try gradually to execute 'split' so that toes of forward leg, in alternating movements, are beyond your vision; and backward leg, in alternating movements, likewise."

The Bicycle

Put your feet on the pedals to cycle with these steps:

1. Inhale to reach your toes long to the front, down to your bottom, and up to the ceiling, while lengthening your other leg to the ceiling.

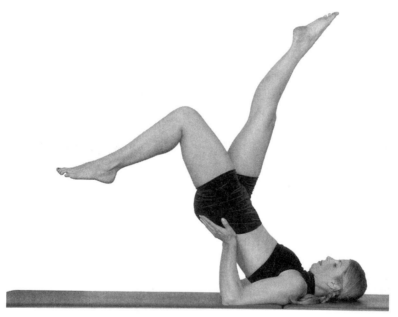

2. Don't drop your knees into your face—lengthen, scoop, pinch, and stay firm. Imagine big cycles as you re-create the motion with your legs.

3. When your leg reaches the ceiling, exhale and start cycling the other leg. Repeat three cycles and then reverse the cycle.

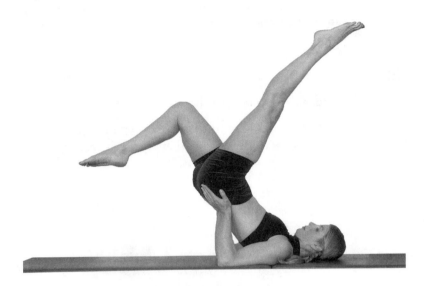

Let's Dance: Can-Can to Hip Circles

Get ready to Can-Can. After that, you can advance to Hip Circles. The focus is on deep abdominal strength, and it's the ultimate love-handle trimmer. In the Can-Can, you're honing your coordination skills, which will come in handy as you progress to Hip Circles.

If you have any back problems, don't progress to Hip Circles. The Can-Can is a safe and fun alternative. Eventually you can drop the Can-Can if you want. For example, after the Teaser you could go right into Hip Circles.

The Can-Can

Create the Can-Can with these steps:

1. Sit with your arms behind you, palms on the floor, or bent at your elbows.

2. Pull your knees in to your chest as close as possible. Point your toes and place them on a fixed point on the mat. Anchor your elbows to the mat to prevent your trunk from moving and your shoulders from hunching. As you do the Can-Can, don't move your toes from that spot, and don't let your knees open.

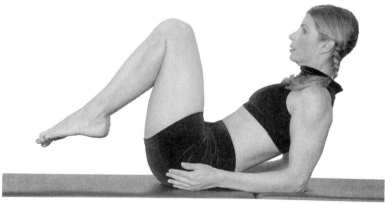

3. Inhale to turn your knees to the right until you're sitting on your hip. Keep your knees stacked directly on top of one another to get the oblique strengthening benefits.

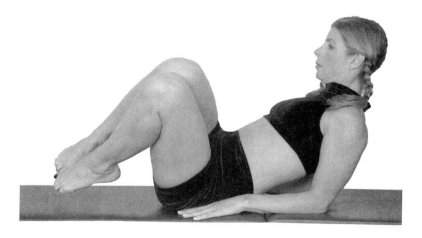

4. Still inhaling, bring your knees to the center and then let them fall to the left. Quickly bring them back through the center to finish on the right side.

5. With your knees bent on your right side, exhale to reach your legs long to the ceiling, leading with your toes on your outside leg. Start left on the next sequence. Repeat three to five times.

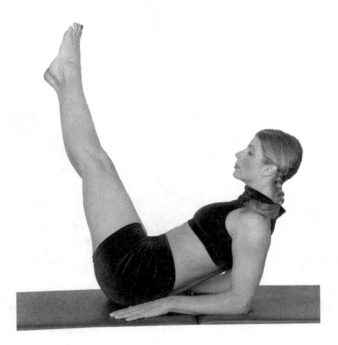

Hip Circles

When practicing Hip Circles, start small and be careful. The weight of your legs can pull your back into an arch. You can also hold on to something (as shown in the photos) to help stabilize your torso. Your legs ultimately will reach out to the floor and then up, without arching your back. This takes a lot of powerhouse strength and lots of coordination.

Upgrade to Hip Circles with these steps:

1. Sit with your arms behind you, palms down, or hold something. Your arms stabilize your trunk, as does your powerhouse.

2. Bend your knees to your chest to lift your toes to the ceiling, and reach out of your hips.

3. Inhale to lower your legs to the left, down to the mat—if possible, exhale to swing your legs up to the ceiling. Don't let your legs open—glue your ankles and knees together. You're drawing a circle on the wall in front of you; however, it doesn't have to be a big circle.

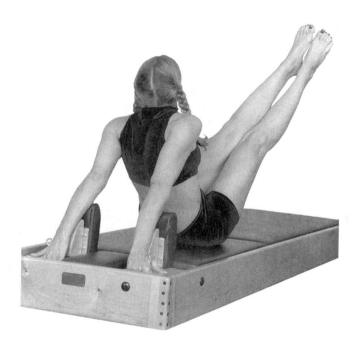

4. Reverse the direction. Repeat three to five times.

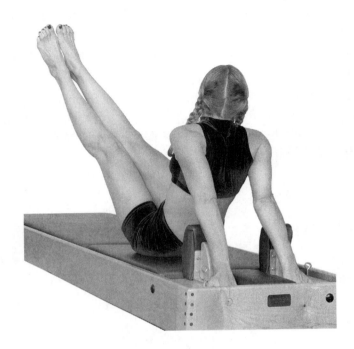

Precision Lifts: Kneeling Side Kicks, the Mermaid, and the Twist

This series is a long yet very beautiful set of moves. It starts with Leg Pull Back, which then transitions into Kneeling Side Kicks. After that, you'll stretch with the Mermaid. Then you'll straighten your legs for the Twist. Whoa! You definitely have your fat-burning work cut out for you—but it's a lot of fun. The sequence flows to strengthen your bod!

Like all the exercises, these moves combine balance, strength, flexibility, and more strength. Yes, stretching, too.

Kneeling Side Kicks

Let's start with Kneeling Side Kicks. Focus on your waistline and hips. The goal is to stay firm in your core and let your legs do all the work. If you feel extremely wobbly, don't kick. Just do the stability work and progress to kicking. In any event, start off with small kicks and make them bigger as your balance improves.

Perfect the Kneeling Side Kicks with these steps:

1. From the Leg Pull Back, bend your left knee while placing the palm of your hand onto the mat directly under your shoulder.

2. Push yourself up and lengthen your top leg out to the side.

3. Lift your leg so it's in line with your hips.

4. Scoop to establish a good base of support between your knee and the palm of your hand.

5. Place your top hand behind your head so your elbow points to the ceiling to open your chest and shoulders.

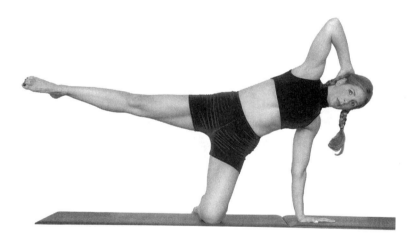

6. Inhale to kick to the front wall. Try to keep your leg at hip height.

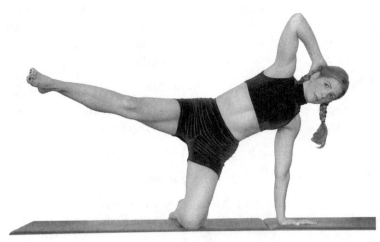

7. Exhale to kick to the back wall, moving nothing except your leg. Don't sink your head and neck into your shoulders as you kick. Keep firm in your belly and stay lifted in your waist.

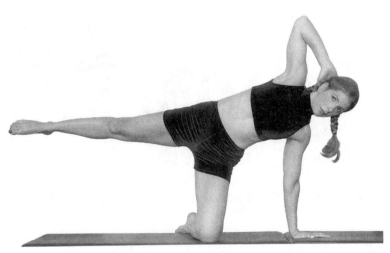

8. After you complete four sets of kicks, drop your leg to the mat, come back to the center, and do the other leg.

Pure Stretch: The Mermaid

Do the Mermaid with flowing arms and breaths. You're soothing your lateral spine or the sides of your body with this stretch.

Stretch with the Mermaid using these steps:

1. Sit on the mat.

2. Bend your knees and shift your weight so your legs are underneath your derriere and you end up sitting on your left hip. Your right knee is on top of your left.

3. With grace, lift your left arm against your face in front of your ear to the ceiling. Keep your right hand on the mat or hold your ankle.

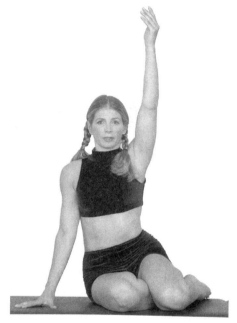

4. Inhale to lift up and over your head to the right, stretching your left side. Exhale to center.

5. With one graceful motion, exhale to switch hands, and lift up and over to stretch your right side.

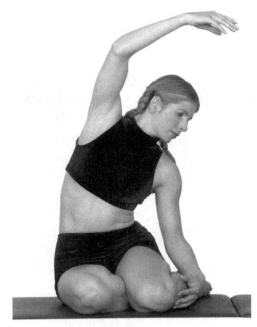

6. Repeat three times and then switch legs.

The Twist

The Twist is a pure power move to strengthen your deep waist oblique muscles and test your balance and control. The goal is to stay absolutely still as you twist. If you can't, just lift and lower your body to build stability. Then progress to the actual Twist.

Test your Twist with these steps:

1. Sit on the mat with your legs out to the side and cross your top foot in front of your back foot.

2. Press the palm of your hand into the mat. Rest your other hand in front of your thighs. Scoop.

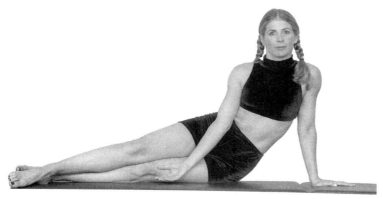

3. Inhale to lift your hips off the mat, anchoring the palm of your hand directly under your shoulder while your other hand reaches over your head. Your upper arm is by your ear as you look at the floor in a straight line from your toes to your fingertips.

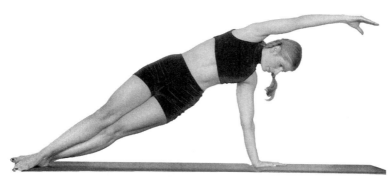

4. Engage the muscles underneath your armpits to stabilize your shoulder and reduce the pressure in your supporting wrist and your body weight traveling toward your feet.

5. Remain firm as you exhale to lower your top hand as you sweep the floor, under your torso.

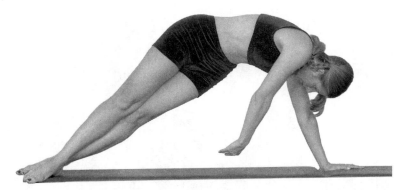

6. Inhale to twist back to open your chest while your top hand reaches back. Look up at the ceiling. The Twist is in your torso, not your legs. Imagine your pelvis is the wheel that rotates your body around. Don't move or sink into your hips—stay firm. Exhale to lower your hips. Repeat twice.

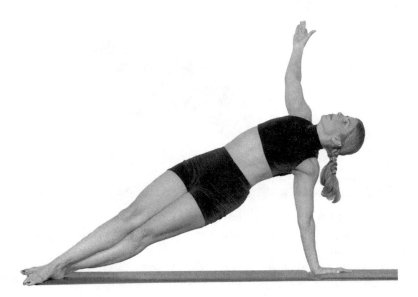

FIT FACT

This exercise is an example of perfect opposition. Your arms and upper body work toward your feet, and your feet work toward your upper body to create a lift in the center so you go up, not sink your body weight into your joints.

Balance in Motion: The Boomerang

Here's a story of a lovely lady who waits patiently for her prince charming. He shows up donning a beloved bow and arrow. After seeing this lovely lady, he imagines her belly button is great for target practice. So he fires and the arrow pierces her belly button, forcing the lady to scoop as she plunges back into the Boomerang.

The Boomerang is a perfect blend of balance, poise, strength, and flexibility, and it works almost every muscle in your body. But you must scoop, scoop, and scoop to balance your body in motion.

Embrace the Boomerang with these steps:

1. Sit tall, with your legs straight in front of you.

2. Place your hands at your sides, palms down into the mat. Cross your right ankle on top of your left ankle.

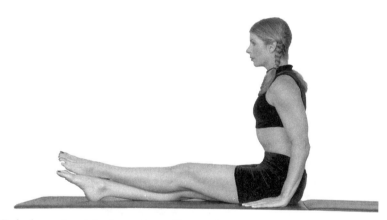

3. Inhale and, with the palms of your hands, lift your legs off the mat to roll over, balancing the weight on your shoulders, not your neck. Your fingertips should reach long along the mat.

4. Exhale to recross your legs quickly; your right ankle uncrosses so your left ankle crosses on top of your right.

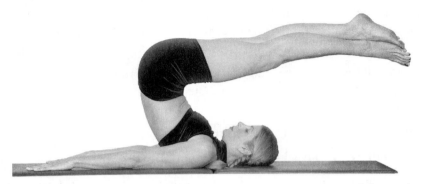

5. Inhale to slide the palms of your hands along the mat to lift you into a Teaser, or V position. Scoop, scoop, scoop.

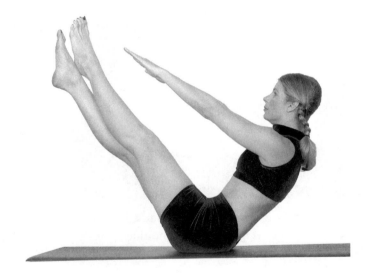

6. Exhale slowly as you balance, circle your arms down by your sides to lower part of your back, clasp your fingers, and reach your hands away from your body. Don't lose your scoop. Stay as still as possible while opening your chest to feel a slight stretch.

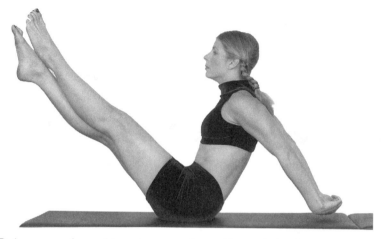

7. Raise your clasped hands up to the ceiling while slowly lowering your legs to the floor with absolute control. No plopping!

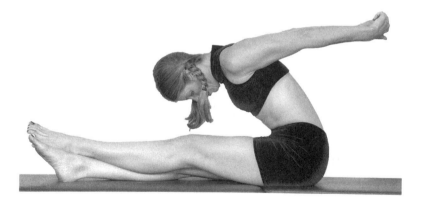

8. Unclasp your fingers, and circle your arms in front, reaching to your toes. Keep scooping, even as you stretch. Your left leg is now on top and ready to boomerang again.

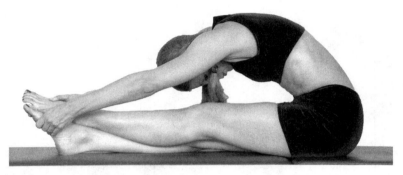

9. After two complete sets, you're ready to bark like a Seal ….

Last Call

Congratulations! This chapter completes the Mat exercises. As you've seen, the Mat requires a lot of practice, as well as focus, concentration, and precision. Remember, the Mat is just one part of Joseph Pilates' methods. There are the machines, too.

This journey is just the beginning to help you get in touch with your body and mind. In this case, practice makes perfect. After a few months, you'll feel more confident, have less flab, and double your core strength.

Be proud because your total look will only get better as you continue to reshape from within.

The Least You Need to Know

- Breathing helps you concentrate and focus.
- Imagery is seeing the exercise in your mind.
- If you can see it, your body will do it.
- Don't do the Leg Pull Front, Leg Pull Back, Kneeling Side Kick, or Twist if you have wrist problems.
- Every move is a delicate mix of balance, control, flexibility, and strength.

The Anticellulite Solution

In This Chapter

- Say good-bye to cellulite
- Legs to die for
- Firm up your bottom
- Still working the powerhouse

Does your butt have too much wiggle? Or a droop in need of a lift? Do your legs jiggle like Jell-O? If so, it's time to de-dimple and de-droop your derriere. No, a random dimple won't kill you, but those dimples should be reserved for the cheeks on your face!

You can tighten these areas with the Side-Kick Series. Imagine a crusade against the unmanageable dimple—you won't have to feel defeated by the battle of dimples and saddlebags ever again! This chapter is the anticellulite solution so you can reshape your backside for good.

De-Fat Your Dimples

To sculpt your bottom half, you need to target the muscles that betrayed you—the muscles that got soft! The Side-Kick Series targets the muscles in your legs and derriere, plus your powerhouse. It's your powerhouse that stabilizes your torso so you can move your legs.

All along you've been pinching your butt cheeks, lifting through the backs of your upper thighs, and scooping your transverse to your spine. Don't stop. The core concepts still apply here. It's these muscles—the pelvic floor muscles, your inner thighs, your hamstrings, and your lower abs—that help stabilize your pelvis as your legs move. Still, you'll also sculpt many muscles you're probably already familiar with: your quadriceps, which run down your thigh, and your hamstrings, which travel from your buttocks to the back of your knee.

Then there are smaller but not forgotten muscles: the *gluteus medius* and *minimus*. These muscles are strategically located on the outside of your thigh to work in harmony with your *gluteus maximus*. Slide your hand down the inside of your thigh. This group of muscles is called the *hip adductors*, while the muscles that run down the outside part of your leg are *hip abductors*, a.k.a. saddlebags.

Empowering Your Patootie

You'll start your legs off easy. In weeks 1 and 2, you'll do three exercises: the Side Kick, the Beat-Beat Up, and the Passé. As the weeks continue, the degree of difficulty will increase. In weeks 3 and 4, you'll challenge your core even more and work your leg muscles with more exercises that use a larger range of motion. And then in weeks 5 and 6, you'll add the most advanced moves to engage even more muscle fibers. Translation: tighter results.

FIT FACT

How many words can you come up with to describe your buttocks? There's *butt, butt cheeks, derriere, heinie, behind, posterior, glutes, rear end, fanny, cheeky, backside, maximus, tail, rump, bottom, tush,* and *tuckus!*

Follow the directions that accompany these movements because they tell you when to add these exercises to your existing Mat routine. Remember, you're adding in exercises as the weeks go on. The Mat exercise Teaser will always follow the Side-Kick Series.

Don't stop between leg exercises. The Side-Kick Series was designed to rap-tap-tap along at a rhythmic pace. The series was brilliantly masterminded to gradually increase the workload so you can transform those stubborn dimples.

The Side-Kick Series is as follows:

- Side Kicks
- Beat-Beat Up
- Side Passé
- Small Circles, Front and Back
- Parallel Leg

- Double-Leg Lift
- Close the Hatch
- Inner Thigh Circles
- Flutter Kicks (small, medium, big)
- Hot Potato
- Grand Ronde de Jambe
- Bicycle (transition)
- Beats on the Belly (transition)

Stay Square

To de-dimple this area, you need to focus on the pinch and scoop in conjunction to work your legs and derriere. In other words, don't flab your tummy; it can't hang over your waistband.

The body position for the Side-Kick Series stays the same as you work from move to move. Here's the important part: keep your hips stacked on top of each other and stay square. The feeling is that your top leg is slightly heavier than your bottom leg, so your upper inner thighs shave past one another. Your knees slightly turn out as if you were in the Pilates V. For example, turn your knee slightly to face the ceiling, leading from your hip joint, while your bottom knee turns down slightly to face the floor.

Square off your shoulders as well. At first, you may feel wobbly as you kick, circle, and bend your leg. Staying square in your upper body as well helps stabilize your torso. Keep in mind that when you're working your legs, your trunk must remain still. You can use your hand for additional support.

You'll start in the beginner/intermediate position. If you have a neck or shoulder injury, lower your bottom hand to the floor so you can rest your head. You can also put a small pad between your support hand and your head or whatever feels comfortable so you don't strain your neck.

PILATES PRECAUTION

The most common mistake students make is they forget to press the palm of their top hand into the mat, so their trunk wobbles and teeters as the leg swings back and forth, throwing off body alignment. In the end, they work the muscles incorrectly, work into the joints, or create muscle imbalances. Use the palm of your top hand for support like a bicycle uses a kickstand.

Strike a pose with this picture:

1. Lie in a straight line, with your neck, shoulders, hips, and legs in line.

2. Use your arm on the mat to support your head, specifically the palm of your hand. Your top hand acts like a kickstand, providing support as your leg moves.

3. Press the palm of your hand into the mat, and activate your triceps to help stabilize you along with your powerhouse.

4. When you're in position, lift your legs to the front of your body at about a 45-degree angle. Your bottom leg reaches long, leading with your toes; turn them under. Your top foot is in a soft point.

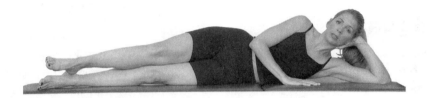

PILATES PRECAUTION

Even though you'll see breathing directions, don't worry if you can't follow the patterns. The important point is to just breathe, never holding your breath.

Off to Get a Better Butt: Weeks 1 and 2

In weeks 1 and 2, you'll perform three exercises: Side Kicks, Beat-Beat Up, Side Passé. And of course, the Mat wouldn't be a workout if you didn't flow with a transition, so Beats on the Belly it is. Think Dorothy in *The Wizard of Oz*. She wanted to go home so badly she clicked her heels together. Instead of seeing the wizard, you're off to get a tighter tush. So click, click, click.

Be careful: you may shock muscles that have been comatose until now. If you feel any burn or pain, do one more and stop. No need to push yourself into a burn—less is always best. Don't forget to complete the Side-Kick Series on the other leg.

Here's the rundown on the working muscles: Side Kicks work your inner and outer thighs, plus gradually warm up your hip joints for more work to come. For example, Beat-Beat Up is a killer for your inner thighs; it stretches and flexes yet doesn't neglect your hips and butt. And then you finish with the Passé; it, too, works all the right places: hips, inner thighs, and butt.

Side Kicks

Let's start with the Side Kicks using these steps:

1. Get in position. Lift your top leg to hip height and slightly turn up your knee, leading from the hip joint.

2. Inhale and, with your hips stacked, swing your leg forward, and pulse two times. The rhythm is kick, and then another small kick. A common mistake is to roll your hips forward as your leg swings, but keep your hips stacked.

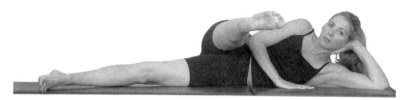

3. Exhale to swing your leg back, adding a small kick. Feel your bottom work, especially as you pulse on the second small kick. Watch out—your back may arch and your ribs may flare out as the weight of your leg swings back. Keep your ribs down and your hips stacked. After six to eight sets, put your heels together, as if they're kissing.

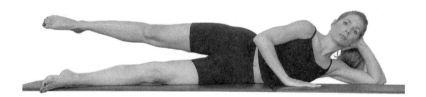

Beat-Beat Up

Follow with Beat-Beat Up in these steps:

1. Inhale and lift your leg up to the ceiling; your knee leads the way. (You can add the beats later, if you want.)

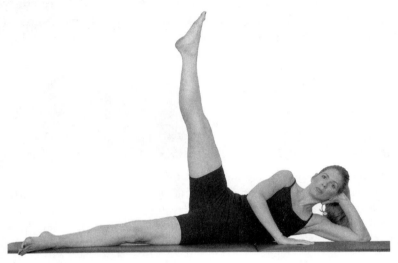

2. Exhale to lower your top heel to your bottom heel, and pulse your heel quickly in front of the foot resting on the mat and in back. Add some self-resistance as you lower to beat-beat. Here's the rhythm: beat-beat—UP! beat-beat—UP! Repeat this six times and seal it with a kiss—heels together.

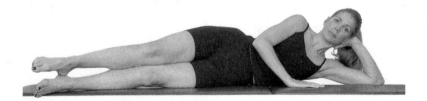

Side Passé

There's no pausing here—go into Side Passé by following these steps:

1. Inhale and slide your heel along the inside of your bottom leg, exposing your inner thigh the whole time.

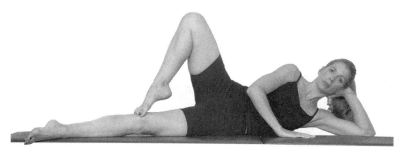

2. Keep inhaling as you bend your knee and lengthen your leg to the ceiling.

3. Exhale and press the top heel to the bottom heel, saying, "One, two, three miles longer …." Bring your top leg down longer than your bottom heel to create length. Repeat three times, and then reverse the direction of the Passé.

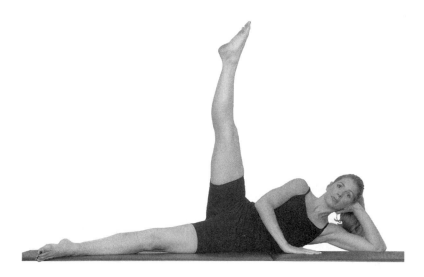

FIT FACT

The most important thing about the Side-Kick Series is to keep your upper body completely still as your leg kicks, circles, and bends. To do this, you must scoop, pinch, and stay square in your hips and shoulders.

Beats on the Belly

Finish with Beats on the Belly:

1. As gracefully as possible, roll onto your belly.

2. Rest your head on your forearms in front of you. Lift your belly button to your spine. Put a $1,000 bill between your butt cheeks. Lift your legs off the mat, about 2 or 3 inches.

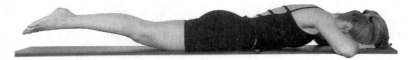

3. Inhale to beat your heels together, counting to five.

4. Exhale while still beating your heels for another set of five.

5. Take a few seconds to rest in Child's Pose (see Chapter 7). Then complete these exercises on the other leg.

Bye, Bye, Butt Rut: Weeks 3 and 4

Let's target your hot spots: your patootie, thighs, and inner thighs. In these weeks, you'll add leg moves that challenge the core even more and increase the range of motion. The Side-Kick Series gets harder and longer. Pay attention to how your body feels. Push it, but don't overdo it.

Focus on keeping your hips stacked. Watch for sloppiness. As the moves increase in difficulty, your body might sacrifice good form for bad form: sinking into your waist, lowering your shoulders, twisting your torso, or just working your leg incorrectly. Sloppiness always coexists with fatigue. Don't complete the set if you can't stay aligned.

FIT FACT

In every exercise, you're strengthening and lengthening while developing coordination and control.

Remember, the leg work is rhythmic—no stopping. In these weeks, you'll add Small Circles, Parallel Leg, Double-Leg Lift, Close the Hatch, Inner Thigh Circles, and Flutter Kicks. The transition is the same, Beats on the Belly.

Small Circles

Start with the Small Circles, Front and Back:

1. From the Side Passé, lengthen your leg to your top heel as if it is working beyond the other heel, pulling from your waistline, knee facing up.

2. Lift your leg just about an inch. Keep the circles small so your inner thighs shave one another.

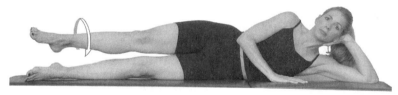

3. Circle the leg five times, touching your heel with every circle. Work from your inner thigh down. In fact, try to touch your thighs—let no light in, so pinch your butt cheeks.

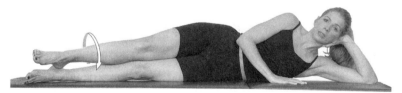

4. Reverse the circles for another 5, totaling 10 small circles.

5. Move your top leg so it reaches back, and keep your hips square. Circle 5 times, and reverse for 5 more, totaling 10 small circles. Breathe normally. Keep your leg back.

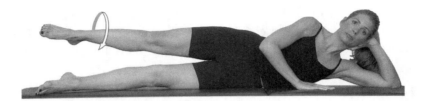

 FIT FACT

Stay lifted from the top of your head to the top of your big toe. Think tall—6 feet tall to create length. Don't sink into your waist, lean back into your hips, or round your shoulders as you bend or kick. Stay square so your legs get the workout they deserve.

Parallel Leg

Next up is Parallel Leg. Follow these steps:

1. Flex your foot to work your leg in parallel. Be sure your hips are stacked.

2. Inhale to lift your leg in three counts—a little higher each time.

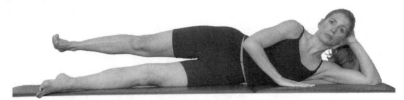

3. Exhale to lower your leg in one count, as if the elevator just fell to the floor, squeezing your inner thighs. Repeat four times.

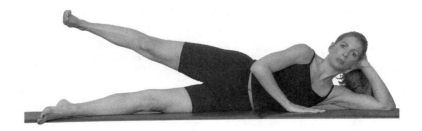

Double-Leg Lift

Next you'll do a Double-Leg Lift, using these steps:

1. Lower your head to the floor to rest on your arm.

2. Straighten your legs so your body is in one straight line from head to toe.

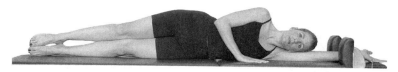

3. Inhale to lift your belly button to your spine and lift your legs off the mat, keeping your knees and ankles together so no light shines through.

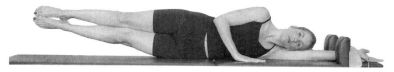

4. Exhale to lower your legs. Repeat four times. On the fourth lift, drop your bottom straight leg to continue with Close the Hatch.

 FIT FACT

To get the most stretch possible, lengthen your legs away from your waist when they're straight. Imagine your legs starting from your belly button.

Close the Hatch

Follow the Double-Leg Lift with Close the Hatch:

1. With split legs, Close the Hatch by lifting and lowering your bottom leg to your top leg.

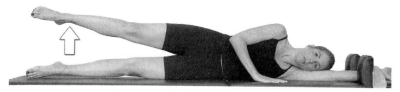

2. Lead from your inner thigh on down. Breathe normally. Repeat five times and then add Inner Thigh Circles.

Inner Thigh Circles

Here's how to do Inner Thigh Circles:

1. With split legs, circle your bottom leg, leading from your inner thigh, touching your heel every time. The rhythm is this: circle 1, touch heel; circle 2, touch heel.

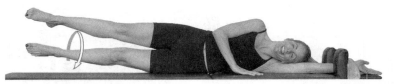

2. Repeat three circles, and reverse the circle for three more, totaling six. Breathe normally. Then lower your legs to just about an inch off the mat for Flutter Kicks.

Flutter Kicks

Put on the finishing touches with Flutter Kicks:

1. Squeeze your butt cheeks, and press the palm of your hand into the mat to stabilize your torso. Nothing moves but your legs; it's a great butt move! Breathe normally.

2. Scissor your legs, making your scissors bigger and bigger.

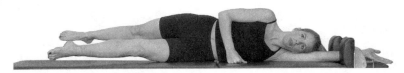

3. Do about 10 flutters. Then you're ready to roll on your belly for Beats on the Belly.

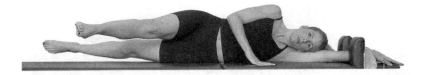

Giving Up Your Rear: Weeks 5 and 6

Worried about your butt? Don't be. It's covered with these exercises, *Grande Ronde de Jambe* and Hot Potato. These moves are the quickest way to redefine your bottom because the exercises require big leg movements and powerhouse power. You're working to stabilize your torso as the movements in your legs get big, bigger, and biggest. Hot Potato, my favorite, will definitely wake up your duff. Pay attention because you may find that the big movements are throwing off your base of support.

> **DEFINITION**
>
> In French, **Grande Ronde de Jambe** means "big leg circles." *Grande Ronde* translates to "big circle" while *de Jambe* means "of the leg."

This exercise completes the Side-Kick Series. As you've been doing, follow the leg work sequence in order, one right after the other. There's one exception: you can replace Beats on the Belly with a new transition, the Bicycle. It's a complete leg stretch: quadriceps, hamstrings, lower back, and all the maximuses.

Here's the rhythm: after Flutter Kick, you'll be in a straight line. Reposition your legs to a 45-degree angle to complete Hot Potato and Grande Ronde de Jambe. Then you'll finish with a thorough leg and hip stretch with the Bicycle.

Hot Potato

Do the Hot Potato using these steps:

1. Imagine your big toe is touching a hot grill. You won't stay there long, so as your toe taps, lift your heel to the ceiling, staying square in your hips. Easy enough—don't forget to breathe normally.

2. Tap your big toe five times, in front.

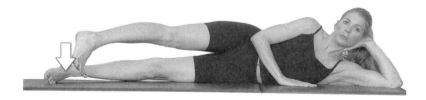

3. On the fifth leg lift, your toe taps behind your supporting leg, near the heel of your bottom foot.

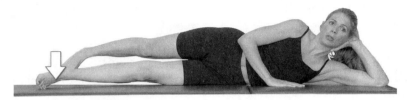

4. Lift and lower five more taps to the back. On the fifth lift, your toe taps front.

5. Tap three more and then behind for three more. Here's the hot, hot, hot part: on the third set, tap front, lift up, pause, and then tap back, lift up, and pause only one time. The Hot Potato order is 5-5, 3-3, 1-1.

Grande Ronde de Jambe

Challenge your thighs with Grande Ronde de Jambe:

1. Lift your top leg so it's at hip height.

2. Swing your leg to the front so you can look at your knee.

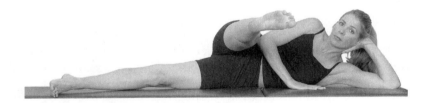

3. Watch your knee as your leg circles to the ceiling. Here's a tip: as your leg circles front and up, keep your knee up the whole time!

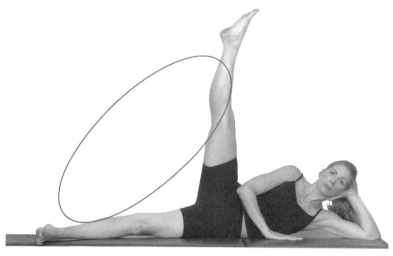

4. Rotate your leg to the back so your knee is in line with your belly button. This rotation comes from your hip socket. Be careful, though. The weight of your leg may pull your hips back. Stay square, and press that top hip into the bottom hip as your leg swings.

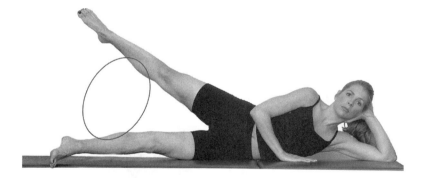

5. Your leg swings down to finish the circle, sweeping past your heels to keep the flow.

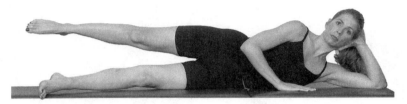

6. Circle three times, breathing normally. Then reverse the pattern: swing your leg back up, to turn in your hip socket and around to the front, pressing your hips square to counterbalance the weight of your leg.

FIT FACT

The big leg circles are a challenge for many students. The most common mistakes are the hips sinking and the waist collapsing as the leg circles. Resist this urge by pulling out of your head and waist and keeping your ribs in.

Bicycle

Finish with the Bicycle:

1. Lift your top arm out by your head, and hold it there.

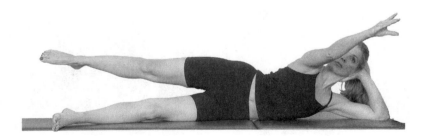

2. Kick your top leg to your arm.

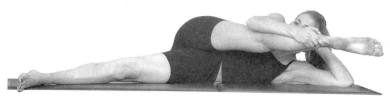

3. Bend your knee and bring it into your chest, as if to kiss your knee.

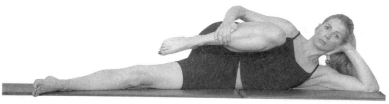

4. With your knee bent, bring it back so your heel touches your belly button. Don't lift any higher than your hip.

5. Reach your bent knee to the back while reaching your top arm long, stretching from your fingertips to your toes.

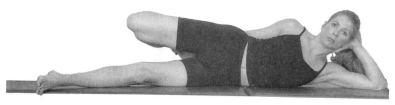

6. Repeat the cycle three times and then reverse it. Keep the movement slow so you feel each stretch. Breathe normally.

After six cycles, continue the Side-Kick Series on your other leg. Then it's time for the Teaser.

Boosting Your Bottom Line

Can you alter your backside? After all, the shape of your patootie was chosen long before you donned a diaper—it's called heredity. No matter what your God-given right, you can shift what you were born with. A healthful diet and these moves can make the most of what you've got. Your goal is to pass the "I can't hold a pencil between my butt cheeks and leg crease" test. In other words, be proud that the pencil drops to the floor! You're on your way to boosting your patootie, derriere, fanny, or my grandmother's favorite—tuckus!

The Least You Need to Know

- Muscle takes up less space than fat. As you develop muscle, you'll get more compact, reshaping your backside for good.
- The Side-Kick Series is made up of 11 exercises that de-dimple your bottom and shrink your saddlebags.
- The important part is to keep your hips stacked on top of each other and stay square during all the leg work so you don't work the wrong muscles.
- Stay lifted from the top of your head to the top of your big toe. Think tall—6 feet tall, to create length. Don't sink into your waist or lean back into your hips, and don't round your shoulders.

Flexing Muscles

In This Chapter

- All about stiff necks
- Tension tamers
- Upper-body, belly, and leg exercises

Whittle away your waddle. You know, the flabby skin that waddles long after you've lifted your arm to, let's say, wave good-bye—it just keeps jiggling and jiggling …. You can have the arms you so deserve. The exercises in this chapter roll into one: sleek arms, strong back, flat abs, and lean legs. How? While toning your arms, you still focus on your powerhouse and legs.

Not only will you look good, but well-toned arms also can protect you from upper-body strain, including your back and neck. You'll lift heavy shopping packages, you'll twist to hoist your child from the floor, and you'll sit hunched at a computer all day multitasking—type, talk, and twist.

What makes lifting, typing, and twisting a breeze? Toned, jiggle-free arms. The good news is that arms respond to exercise super-fast. The muscle groups in your arms are smaller than your thighs—and for most of us, there's less fat that wobbles. So you'll see results fairly quickly.

Dust off your dumbbells, because you're about to use them to super-sculpt your arms and upper back. These exercises target all the right muscles: deltoids, rhomboids, latissimus, trapezius, biceps, and triceps, not to mention the smaller muscle groups that enhance your posture. So get ready to get jiggle free!

To Tense or Not to Tense?

What's the long-term result of overtensing your muscles? Dysfunctional muscles due to a buildup of lactic acid in the muscle fibers. Lactic acid is a waste product of working muscles, which dissipates as the muscle rests. However, let's say your muscles are always tense—turned on and overworked.

Then the problem is twofold. When muscles are always working, you can usually feel the effects before the results. You might be sore and stiff. However, there's a silent enemy within. If your muscles don't relax—let's say because you're constantly tensed—then lactic acid also builds.

Whatever the case, an accumulation of lactic acid can cause injury to the tissue. Injuries to the muscles can compromise the way they respond. For example, a muscle might not be able to reach its normal length; it has shortened, and so has your movement. Is this a problem? You bet. The body is a closed system, lining up from the head, neck, shoulders, hips, knees, and feet. If one part is misaligned, that means trouble for the rest of the body. The body will do anything to work as naturally as possible, even if that means sacrificing other muscle groups to compensate. Constriction throws off the body's natural rhythm.

We hold most of our tension in our neck, shoulders, and upper back. The upper trapezius (or traps, for short), then, is the most overused muscle. Not only do we tense up for the day-to-day stress, but we also spend most of the day hunched over a desk or lifting heavy objects. As the upper trapezius overworks, the lower traps are underused; weak arms compound the problem. After all, if you don't have the arm strength, either your neck or your back will pick up the slack, and an overused upper back results in an aching back.

If you can recognize and let go of tension in your upper traps, you're working toward releasing it. You can save a lot of wasted energy that can be put to better use. Many of these exercises can help, too. Think about keeping your shoulders back and down; hang your shoulders, and keep your pits to your hips to unglue your shoulders from your ears. Besides reinforcing good body alignment, you're not creating any extra stress in your upper back, which needs no extra stress.

My Stiff Neck

So you're desk-bound and your neck aches. How are you holding your head? Does it hang forward? Overworked, overstressed, and fatigued upper traps eventually can cause you to hang your head slightly forward. After all, if the muscle can't function wholly, it can't hold your body correctly.

The key is not to forget your neck muscles. The major ones are the *upper trapezius,* the *levator scapulae,* and the *sternocleidomastoid.* The upper trap runs from the base of your skull past your scapula. The levator scapulae starts just below the back of your skull as well and ends at your scapula. The muscle in front is the sternocleidomastoid; it attaches to two bones, the breast bone and collarbone. This thick muscle lifts your chin to your chest and moves your head from side to side.

DEFINITION

There are three major neck muscles. The **upper trapezius** runs from the base of the skull past the scapula, the **levator scapulae** starts just below the back of the skull and ends at the scapula, and the **sternocleidomastoid** attaches to two bones in the front of your body, the breast bone and the clavicle.

A stiff neck boils down to stress and weak neck muscles. Toned and flexible neck muscles help keep your head in its right place, which is directly over your shoulders. So if you spend your day leaning over a desk, stretch your neck muscles every hour. And find ways to tame your tension. Take a stress-management class or practice breathing techniques. Finally, you've got to strengthen these muscles!

So you've got to figure out a way to combat the stress and strengthen and stretch the muscles in your neck as well as your upper back. Easy enough.

Muscle, Not Momentum!

Okay, your upper-back muscles are overworked, but how are the joints in your shoulders affected? After all, toned muscles protect the joints. The shoulder joint has an unusual anatomical structure; it's geared to give you a wide range of motion and greater flexibility. You can weight-train to reach for a crying baby or to lift heavy boxes.

We use our arms so frequently we often take them for granted, until we feel a little twinge in the shoulder. What's going on? Pent-up tension, lack of flexibility and strength, along with rapid sloppy movements make this joint susceptible to injury.

If a muscle is constricted, it can't enjoy a full range of movement and flexibility. If it's weak, another muscle will compensate. If it's sloppy and fast in movements, eventually the muscle will give out. You'll always come back to the guiding principles: smooth, controlled movement is more effective and less stressful on the joints than a wild, uncontrolled, large movement. In other words, use the muscle, not momentum.

The shoulder girdle is a complex combination of ligaments, tendons, and muscles that protect a group of joints. It's a good size, starting with the clavicle, the shoulder blades, the upper-arm bones, and the rib cage. The primary function is to connect the arms to the trunk. Your shoulder girdle is held in place by muscles and gets its strength from muscles, which is why you must work the muscles evenly and correctly. For example, you don't want to lift weight if your shoulders are glued to your ears.

As you know, there are deep stabilizing muscles as well as movement muscles. The deep rotator cuff muscles—the *subscapularis, supraspinatus, infraspinatus*, and *teres minor*—give stability to the shoulders. These muscles encircle the shoulder joint; you can feel them rotating your shoulders in and out. With strong rotators, the large muscle movers can do their job with ease and without injury.

DEFINITION

The shoulder girdle is stabilized by a group of muscles called the rotator cuff, or shoulder rotators. These muscles—the **subscapularis, supraspinatus, infraspinatus,** and **teres minor**—encircle the shoulder joint so the large movement muscles can move with ease.

Major movement muscles of the arm include the biceps and triceps. It's easy to train your biceps because they're sitting on the top portion of your arm. Now feel the muscle in the back of your arm. That's the triceps group. We often neglect them, and for that reason these are the first to turn flabby. The flab waves long after you're done saying good-bye!

The other muscles include the shoulder muscles or deltoids (delts, for short). Then there are the chest muscles, the pectoralis major and minor. On your back are a few big muscle groups: the trapezius, which is divided into the upper and lower traps; the rhomboids, located between your shoulder blades; the latissimus dorsi, the largest back muscle; and finally, the serratus anterior, the muscle underneath your armpits. Strengthen these muscles evenly, and you're on your way to better posture.

Leaning into the Wind

Just because you're working your arms doesn't mean your abs won't work also. You're aiming for tone in your legs and lots of work in your abs to support your torso. Let go of your tension and unlock your joints. Lengthen your spine, relax your shoulders, and align your neck so it's free and over your shoulders.

To do your standing arm work, find a mirror and then follow these steps:

1. Get in your Pilates V. Remember, your heels are glued together, and your toes are about three fingers apart. Your legs are straight, but your knees are never locked. Balance your weight evenly between your feet.

2. Create a long spine by lengthening out of the top of your head, as if someone has lifted you up by your head. Then scoop your navel to your spine to create a stable center.

3. Imagine the wind blowing in your face—it's hurricane force. To stand tall and stable, you have to lean into the wind and remain rigid from the base of your pelvis to the top of your head, scooping your navel to your spine the whole time while pinching your butt cheeks. Think about putting a $1,000 bill between your cheeks, and squeeze it. The more your powerhouse works, the more stable you will be.

4. Hang your shoulders. Remind yourself over and over again, pits to your hips. But don't pull back your shoulders; it's a natural hang from the shoulder sockets. Don't worry if they naturally hang slightly forward; don't force them back.

5. As you lean into the wind, the tendency is to hang your neck forward, as if you have a dreadful double-chin. Don't. Keep your chin parallel to the floor, and tighten your torso.

After you've mastered leaning into the wind, rise up to your toes, keeping your heels together. That's right, you can do the Arm Series on your toes if you need a little extra oomph, lowering your heels on the last exercise. Besides getting a great workout, you're building your balance.

Jiggle Free: The Standing Arms Series

Do the Standing Arms Series at the beginning or end of your Mat workout. Anyone can do this series, and all you need is a pair of 1- to 3-pound dumbbells. This is great for the older set who need to strengthen the upper back or for a pregnant woman who needs pain relief for her aching back.

As with every exercise, you're stabilizing your body against movement. Focus on your shoulder joints—the muscles and your form. Work to tone the muscles around the joint without stressing the joint itself, meaning no momentum. Don't forget about the principle of self-resistance: add resistance in both directions to get the most out of your workout. As always, review your mental checklists along with these directions:

- Pits to your hips; don't force your shoulders back.
- Be sure your shoulders are even; one shoulder shouldn't be higher than the other.
- No tensing anywhere.
- Engage in slow and controlled movements instead of big movements driven by momentum.
- Don't hang your head forward.
- Keep your wrists straight at all times.
- Don't grip your dumbbells. This causes needless tension.

Even if you're sculpting your back to show it off in the hottest halter top, know this: by strengthening your upper back, you'll improve your posture and protect yourself from injury. So follow the directions to do the Standing Arms Series listed here:

- Biceps Curls
- Boxing
- The Fly
- Zip-Ups
- Arm Circles
- Chest Expansion
- Side Stretch

Basic Biceps Curls

Biceps Curls? No brainer, right? However, this exercise is often done incorrectly. Elbows fly, the torso rocks, the shoulders levitate, and the arms swing back and forth. These are all no-nos.

Think stabilization! Work your biceps without jerking your trunk up and down—stay stable. Glue your elbows to your rib cage, press your shoulders to your hips, and slow down to isolate your biceps muscle.

You'll do one set of Biceps Curls and work your powerhouse. You'll curl in what's called the *Pilates box*, meaning your limbs should not work wider than your shoulders and hips.

DEFINITION

The **Pilates box** refers to the area within the boundaries of your torso, no wider than your shoulders and hips.

Do the basic Biceps Curls in these steps:

1. In your Pilates V, extend your arms out in front of you, at shoulder height and with your palms up.

2. Inhale and slowly curl your arms toward your shoulders. Keep your wrists straight, and don't grip the dumbbells.

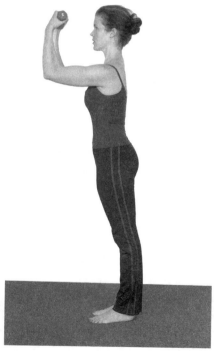

3. Exhale and return your arms to the starting position. Remember, self-resistance! Keep your elbows in place and your shoulders down. You're going for length, so reach your fingertips as far away from your face as possible, self-resisting in both directions. Do 10 reps.

Boxing

For this exercise, you're still incorporating a few muscle groups: your triceps, delts, rotators, and biceps. Let's back up for a second. Think back to your shoulder girdle. Picture your shoulder rotators; they're deep. The deltoid muscles are superficial—you can feel them—and they're divided into three muscles to support the shoulder: front or anterior, middle or medial, and back or posterior. You're working your back deltoid and triceps.

Test your Boxing skills in these steps:

1. Get in a squat position, with your knees in line with your heels and your knees directly beneath your hips.

2. Sit on the back of your heels so you feel the muscles in your legs work. No flab should hang over your waistband. Scoop your navel to the spine.

3. Flatten your back. Look down at the floor so your head is in line with your spine. Dangle your arms in front of you. With your hands palms in, draw your arms to your rib cage, with your elbows glued to your ribs.

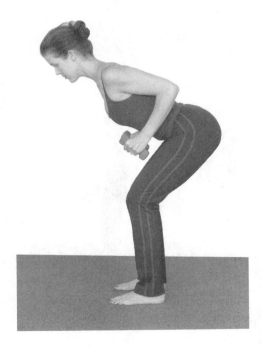

4. Inhale and lift your right arm in front of your body as your left arm extends back. Move within your Pilates box.

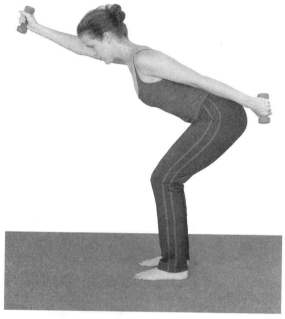

5. Exhale and return to the starting position. Draw your arms to your rib cage, with your elbows shaving your ribs.

6. Inhale and repeat directions as you extend your left arm out while your right arm lengthens back. Do 10 reps.

Develop Your Delts: The Fly

With this exercise, the tendency is to lift higher than your shoulder height. Watch for shoulder unevenness and belly bulge. As you work with a flat back, your tummy may bulge out. Remember, scoop your navel to your spine the whole time. The focus is your rear delts and rhomboid group.

ON THE MAT

Always apply the guiding principles: smooth, controlled movement is more effective and less stressful on the joints than a wild, uncontrolled, large movement. Use muscle, not momentum.

Do the Fly in these steps:

1. Get in a squat position, with your knees in line with your heels and directly beneath your hips.

2. Sit on the back of your heels so you feel the muscles in your legs work. Don't let your flab hang over your waistband. Scoop your navel to your spine.

3. Flatten your back. Look down at the floor so your head and neck are in line with your spine. Dangle your hands in front, palms in.

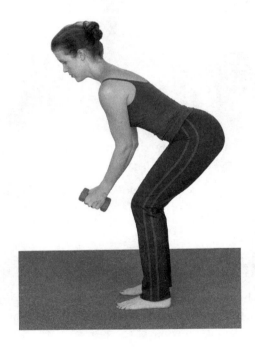

4. Inhale to lift your arms out to the side; keep them even. Crack an imaginary walnut between your shoulder blades to work your rhomboids. Exhale down. Do 10 reps.

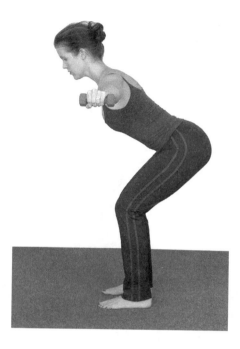

Pump It Up: Zip-Ups

Maybe you've heard of an "upright row." Here's the same exercise, only it's called a Zip-Up. This exercise targets your middle deltoid among other muscles such as your rhomboids, your trapezius, and the upper and back area of your arms.

What makes this exercise a little more difficult is that your shoulders tend to lift with your arms. Focus on stabilizing your shoulders by pressing your shoulders down before lifting.

Do a Zip-Up in these steps:

1. In the Pilates V, drop your hands so they rest in front of your thighs, with your palms down in a narrow grip.

2. Inhale, and bend your elbows to lift the dumbbells following your center line. Imagine zipping up your jeans, and just keep going.

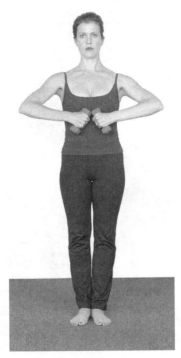

3. Exhale and lower the hands to your pubic bone, resisting gravity on the way down. Do 10 reps.

Stretch, Flex, Go: Arm Circles, Chest Expansion, and Side Stretch

Arm Circles strengthen the smaller muscle groups and arm joints that support the larger shoulder muscles, the rotator group. These circles are a wonderful way to release tension and open your back while toning your chest and shoulders and adding a little definition to your arms.

Make your circles small from your shoulder joints. The sequence is to lift your arms from your thighs to the top of your head following your center line, circling 10 times and inhaling every 3 to 5 counts. Then reverse the circles and exhale on the way down.

> **FIT FACT**
>
> You can always *relevé* to make the exercises a little more challenging. Pretend you're a ballerina and raise up on your toes to initiate the moves. Then press your heels down as you return to the starting position. Or stay up on your toes during the entire set to get maximum work and build your balance.

You'll then finish with two stretches: Chest Expansion and Side Stretch. In Chest Expansion, the focus stretch is your neck and chest muscle groups. Of course, the Side Stretch stretches just that: muscles in your side.

Arm Circles

Circle your arms in these steps:

1. In the Pilates V, lengthen your arms out to the side.

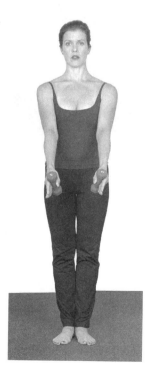

2. Open and widen your upper back to feel the stretch. Relax your neck muscles by maintaining distance between your ears and your shoulders.

3. Keep lengthening your arms away, reaching out to the sides of the room as you circle your arms up over your head and down to your thigh.

4. Inhale, circling up to your head for 10.

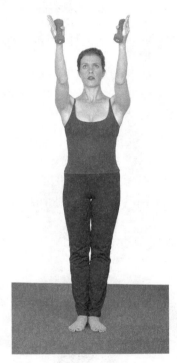

5. Exhale and circle down to your thigh.

Chest Expansion

Stretch with Chest Expansion in these steps:

1. In your Pilates V, extend your arms in front. Slowly inhale and press your arms back, with your palms back, lifting your chest to open it.

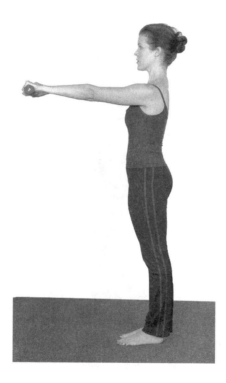

2. Still inhale as you turn your head to the right, to the center, and to the left to stretch your neck and shoulder muscles. Imagine holding on to a set of heavy springs as you press your arms back.

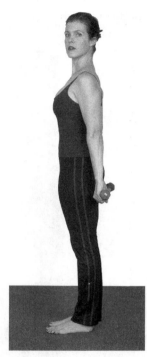

3. Exhale and return your arms to the starting position.

4. Repeat the same directions, but start the neck stretch in the opposite direction: left, center, and right. Do three to five reps.

PILATES PRECAUTION

If you feel any tingling in your fingers, lower your arms and rest before trying again. Build up slowly. If the tingling is troublesome, leave out Arm Circles. You may have some constriction in your muscle that's pressing on a nerve.

Side Stretch

Unbend with Side Stretch in these steps:

1. Inhale your arm up.

2. Exhale over to the side while your right hand reaches down your side.

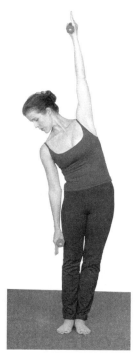

3. Use your powerhouse to control all the movements. Then reverse the directions—inhale to come up, and exhale to stretch over the other side. Do three to five reps.

Minor but Mighty

Yes, your muscles are smaller, but they're important to your frame and sex appeal. These muscles make a big contribution to the stability of the shoulder girdle. Focus on them all to lessen your chances of injury and to keep you looking good!

The Least You Need to Know

- Even though the focus is your upper-body muscles, you'll work your power-house and legs by leaning into the wind.
- When muscles are overworked or tense, there's a buildup of lactic acid.
- Accumulation of lactic acid can injure muscle tissues and restrict movement.
- The only piece of equipment you need for these exercises is a pair of 1- to 3-pound dumbbells.

Glossary

aerobic   Exercises that use oxygen, such as running, walking, and so on.

anaerobic   Exercises that don't use oxygen, such as weight training, sprinting, and so on.

atrophy   The state in which muscles waste away to the point where you can't engage in day-to-day activities. This doesn't happen because of old age, but because of an inactive, sedentary lifestyle.

bone by bone   A phrase that refers to the act of stacking your vertebra one at a time. This core concept is used in almost every exercise, so get used to peeling your spine up and down.

bone in its joint   A phrase that refers to the joint being in its proper place. This proper joint alignment permits the limbs to move safely in a wide variety of movements without wear and tear on the joint. *Bone in its joint* particularly pertains to the ball-and-socket joints of the hips and shoulders. Remember, first you stabilize the body and then you move it!

Chin to Your Chest   The safest position for your head, neck, and back, this position works in line with gravity to hold your head in a safe position.

concentric contraction   A contraction that shortens the muscle.

cross-training   A method of building overall fitness with multiple activities. Complete fitness usually cannot be achieved with just one single sport or activity, so cross-training is a must to prevent injury, burnout, and overtraining, whether mental or physical.

diaphragm   A partition of muscles and tendons in the midriff. When you draw in air, your diaphragm relaxes and moves downward to create a vacuum, sort of like pushing an accordion in and out to generate music. This vacuum draws air into your lungs. To get rid of the air, your diaphragm contracts and rises up to push out all the air from your lungs.

eccentric contraction   A contraction that lengthens the muscle.

Grand Ronde de Jambe   An exercise whose name, in French, actually means "big leg circles."

isometric contraction   A contraction in which the muscle doesn't move when it's contracted.

kyphosis posture   An exaggerated curve in the thoracic spine.

lengthen   The action of "growing yourself tall." This length comes from your spine, as if you're pulled up from the top of your head by a string.

levator scapulae   One of the major neck muscles, it starts just below the back of the skull and ends at the scapula.

lordosis   An exaggeration of the curvature to the lumbar region.

metabolism   How the body burns calories. You can be doing absolutely nothing, and your body will burn calories. You can alter your metabolic rate by increasing your lean muscle mass and reducing your overall fat.

movement muscles   Muscles that tend to be superficial in nature.

neutral pelvis   A position in which the spine is in its natural length, meaning your pelvis does not tilt. To find neutral pelvis on your body, feel the little bony protrusions toward the top of your pelvis, known as the iliac crests. With the heel of your hand, feel your pubic bone. Find the distance between those two points, and lay your hand flat.

peeling your spine off   The action of rolling your back off the mat as if picking up a string of pearls one at a time. The mat or spinal articulation protects your back as you roll up and down, increases the flexibility of your spine, and works the powerhouse.

Pilates box   A term meaning to work within the boundaries of your torso, no wider than your shoulders and hips.

Pilates stance   A stance in which your feet are slightly turned out from the heels so you make a small V. Your feet are no wider than three fingers apart.

Pinch, Lift, and Grow Tall   The length that comes from your spine as your head floats up, lifting every bone. Pinch your butt cheeks so you grow even taller. This position is a neutral pelvis, meaning your pelvis does not tilt.

Pinch, Pinch, Pinch Your Butt Cheeks   A posture in which you imagine a $1,000 bill between your butt cheeks and then squeeze to work all the right areas: your butt cheeks, the upper back of your inner thighs, and the ever-so-vital pelvic floor muscles that keep your internal organs and muscles from dropping out of your body.

powerhouse   Your muscular girdle of strength. The powerhouse sort of looks like a thick rubber band or corset that wraps around the middle part of your body, expanding from the bottom of your rib cage to the line across your hips and wraps around to your back.

pronation   A position in which you turn in your ankles so your body weight is unnaturally displaced on the arches of your feet.

proprioceptive system   Literally "own reception," proprioception coordinates your every movement in time and space.

push from the tush   An action in which you initiate the movement from your bottom: your tush, upper thighs, the back of your upper thighs, and your powerhouse.

scapula stabilization   An action in which you pull your shoulders slightly back and then down, as if your shoulder blades are drawing down your back. Think of the muscles underneath your arms preparing you for the movement—your pits to your hips.

self-talk   Thinking or talking to yourself—a type of internal communication. Use this mental training method to enhance physical performance.

serratus anterior   A broad, thin muscle covering the lateral rib cage and connecting to your shoulder blades. It holds your shoulder blades in place, which helps stabilize your shoulders.

shoulder girdle   The main purpose of the shoulder girdle is to connect your arms to your body. This structure is stabilized by a group of muscles called the rotator cuff, or shoulder rotators. The subscapularis, supraspinatus, infraspinatus, and teres minor encircle the shoulder joint so the large movement muscles can move with ease.

Spine to Mat   A position in which you imagine your torso weighs 50 pounds. It's heavy, and it's anchored to the floor.

stabilizing muscles   Deep muscles hidden between, under, and behind some of the more common muscles. The transverse is a perfect example of a stabilizing muscle.

sternocleidomastoid   A major neck muscle that attaches to two bones in the front of your body, the breast bone and the clavicle.

supination An action in which you roll out your ankles, which could negatively affect your muscle tone and the shape of your legs from your ankles to your hips.

synovial fluid The body's natural version of WD-40 for your joints. When you move, especially in a slow, controlled manner, you're increasing synovial fluid production, whether it's in your spine, hip, shoulder, or some other part of your body. This keeps your joints flexible, protects them from seizing up, and perhaps prevents one of today's most debilitating diseases—arthritis.

theory of opposition This theory moves the body in two different directions to engage more muscle groups. It increases the resistance of all the exercises and gets you in touch with your body.

transversus abdominis The deepest of abdominal muscles, sometimes called the transverse.

upper trapezius A major neck muscle that runs from the base of the skull past the scapula.

visualization The act of strengthening your inner power so you can achieve the results you want. Train your brain, and your body will physically respond.

Index

DISCARD